THE HERBERT
SHELTON READER

The Herbert Shelton Reader

The Development of Disease, Food Combining Made Easy & Principles of Natural Hygiene

by

Herbert Shelton

MOCKINGBIRD
PRESS

Cover Art by Sharon Grey, © 2019 Mockingbird Press
Cover Design by Nami Kurita, © 2020 Mockingbird Press
Book Interior Design by Maria Johnson

Publisher's Cataloging-In-Publication Data

Shelton, Herbert, author
The Herbert Shelton Reader: The Development of Disease, Food Combining Made Ease & Principles of Natural Hygiene / Herbert Shelton

Paperback	ISBN-13: 978-1-953450-09-8
Hardback	ISBN-13: 978-1-953450-10-4
Ebook	ISBN-13: 978-1-953450-11-1

1. Health & Fitness—Naturopathy. 2. Health, Relationships & Personal Development—Mind, Body, Spirit—Complementary Therapies, Healing and Health, I. Herbert Shelton. II. Title. III. The Development of Disease, Food Combining Made Easy & Principles of Natural Hygiene.

HEA016000 / VXHF

Type Set in Schoolbook / **Franklin Gothic Demi**

Mockingbird Press, Augusta, GA
info@mockingbirdpress.com

CONTENTS

FOREWORD

Herbert Shelton was, in many ways, a man ahead of his own time. Born at the close of the 20th century, Shelton was an adherent of the Hygienic movement and a tireless advocate of alternative medicine. Throughout his life he opposed mainstream medical practices; he warned that drugs were being over-prescribed and that hospitalization often made sick patients get sicker. Shelton dedicated his life to offering a different approach to health. He wrote extensively about the benefits of a plant-based diet, the natural healing properties of the body, and the importance of avoiding drugs and surgery.

More than anything else, Shelton emphasized the need to become attuned to the natural processes of the body. He warned that "civilized" man had grown out of touch with the promptings of his own instincts, and that there was an urgent need to reconnect to the physical side of life – to eat nutritious food (raw, when possible), exercise, take in the sun, and get plenty of proper rest. Shelton warned that failing to listen to the body's natural needs could lead to serious disease. But he also believed that at almost any stage, the body could be set back on the right and healthy course.

Herbert Shelton was born in Wylie, Texas on October 6, 1895. A storm was raging on the night of his birth. Baby Herbert was born two months premature, and he was tiny; at birth, he weight less than three pounds and must have seemed very fragile. His parents kept him warm in a make-shift crib fashioned from a cigar box, which they kept by the side of the family's iron stove. The frail baby grew into a strong, robust young man and an avid weight lifter. He took an early interest in nutrition and exercise and read everything he could find on the subject.

Shelton's parents were devout Christians who raised their son with a strong moral compass, a deeply-ingrained sense of self-discipline, and a good command of scripture. Shelton was a pious child, but he eventually moved away from organized religion. Years later, though, even after he had declared himself an agnostic, the influence of his religious upbringing was still evident. Some of his writing has the rolling cadence of Biblical verses. His teachings are full of calls to set aside worldly habits and to pursue a disciplined life. His writing is also full of stories of both human frailty and redemption.

* * *

Shelton's interest in nutrition and natural healing began when he was very young. As a boy, he studied farm animals and noticed the way they all instinctively fasted when they were sick. He also studied the works of health writers like Bernarr McFadden and Russell Trall. In 1921 he married Ida Pape, and the couple moved to New York City so that Shelton could complete his studies. He earned the title of Doctor of Naturopath and went to work as a teacher.

Shelton was always certain that he wanted to work in healthcare, but it took him a little time to find the approach that was just right for him. He spent some years studying different theories before finally deciding that the most meaningful system he had come across was the Hygiene movement. That movement had been launched in 1832 – almost a century before Shelton came across it – by Isaac Jennings and Sylvester Graham. Shelton revered the movement for its focus on maintaining health and vitality, instead of on curing disease. When he was 27, he vowed to revive the movement, writing,

"We will bring clarity out of chaos. I will resuscitate a dying movement. I will rebuild and synthesize the system of Hygiene. Principles that are forgotten will be refurbished. A whole literature will be salvaged. I will fan its glowing embers into a fierce flame." He went on the found the American Natural Hygiene Society and to run a Health School where he educated the public about the Hygiene movement.

* * *

The Hygienist system was highly unorthodox, especially for the early and middle of the twentieth century. Shelton's beliefs put him at odds with the medical community, and, in fact, often landed him in trouble with the law. Fortunately, he was well-equipped by nature to handle hardship for the sake of his beliefs. As a young man, he had been arrested and jailed for opposing World War One. Later in life, after he had become a practicing Naturopath and a member of the Hygienic movement, he was repeatedly arrested for "practicing medicine without a license."

In spite of his troubles with the law, Shelton did gain a sizeable following. People flocked to his Health School and bought his books and magazines. Gandhi invited him to come and spend six months with him in India; unfortunately, World War Two got in the way. In 1956, Shelton was even nominated to run for president, on a third party ticket at the Vegetarian Party Convention in New York. He was no longer an obscure figure, toiling alone. But Shelton's struggles continued.

It was difficult to earn a living as a Naturopath. Shelton, his wife, Ida, and their three children experienced intense and prolonged poverty. Ida, who had great faith in her husband's beliefs, went to work as supplement the family's income, acting as a laundress, a child minder, and whatever else she could do to bring in extra funds. It was a difficult life, and over the years, the Sheltons' marriage felt the strain.

Eventually, the man who had always been the veritable picture of health succumbed to Parkinson's Disease. By 1972, the disease had left Shelton unable to walk or to talk clearly. He spent the next thirteen years bedridden, reduced to dictating instead of writing, and of course, unable to see patients. His followers believed that Shelton had fallen ill because for so many years, he had driven his body and brain too far. Instead of taking regular rest and getting plenty of sleep, as good Hygiene practices suggested, Shelton had worn himself out writing books, delivering lectures, and advising the people who came to him for help. The result was a man who, perhaps, fell ill before his time. However, that same man left the world forty books, countless articles, and a trove of ideas about health and vitality which are still relevant today.

* * *

Herbert Shelton was a prolific writer, and it would be virtually impossible to read all of his works. However, Shelton tended to return again and again to a few major themes, all of which are included in this collection. Those themes include the nature of disease; diet and nutrition; fasting; and the Hygiene movement itself. In many ways, Shelton was concerned with what we might call preventive care today.

Shelton believed that the doctors of his time were looking at the problem of disease backwards. He pointed out that most of the time, doctors don't diagnose a condition until it has reached a very advanced stage. In many cases, he wrote, medical men didn't diagnose the condition until after the patient's death, when an autopsy was performed. To Shelton, this was an absurd situation. As he wrote,

"When a pathological condition becomes manifest so that a diagnosis, right or wrong, may be made, this is not its beginning. Indeed its beginning may be, and often is years prior to this. Its development is invariably slow, gradual, insidious, causing little to no disturbance to the body and no visible sign of its presence."

Shelton's philosophy flipped normal medical practice on its head. Instead of standing by passively and allowing disease to develop, he believed in paying attention to the body's needs at every stage of life. If those needs were met, then disease would never have the chance to take root. "If the pre-clinical stages are prevented the advanced stages won't develop," he wrote.

What allows disease to flourish? Shelton argued that years of living poorly can sap a person's strength, reducing their body's vitality so that it loses its natural power to heal itself. Centuries of civilization have weakened mankind, he believed. He blamed overeating, lack of exercise, too much time spent indoors, and a chronic tendency to worry for most of the ills which plague modern man. He also blamed what he called "stimulants," or caffeine and alcohol, for throwing people's nervous systems off-kilter.

Shelton believed that most diseases were caused by what he called "voluntary habits," or by what we might call "lifestyle choices." He wrote,

"The person who conserves his nervous energies, who does not indulge in excesses and dissipation, who eats sensibly and moderately, who secures plenty of rest and sleep, who takes daily physical exercise, and who secures an abundance of fresh air and sunshine, will not be troubled by catarrh or any other disease."

On one level, Shelton's prescription for a healthy life was simple: eat well and moderately, get plenty of fresh air and exercise, sleep, and don't worry too much. However, his teachings also went into far more detail about proper nutrition. Shelton argued that a good digestion is at the root of good health. In many of his works – including in "Food Combining" – he called for serious changes to the way we eat.

"Food Combining" starts out from the premise that civilized men have lost touch with their instincts and no longer eat correctly. Shelton writes that eating "haphazardly" is the leading cause of digestive inefficiency, causing food to rot, undigested, in the gut before our bodies can use the nutrients it should yield. He warned that eating in a hurry, snatching a few bites on the run, and eating at odd hours was ruining people's digestion. He also cautioned against what we might call "emotional eating" today – eating when not hungry, to cope with one's worries and anxiety.

Shelton advocated eating at regular hours and in careful combinations. ("Food Combinations" sets out his recommendations for which food should be eaten together, and which pairings should be avoided.) For the most part, he said, people should rely on raw fruits and vegetables. Proteins should be included in one's diet, but were not as important as was popularly believed. Shelton warned against what he called the "diet fad" calling for high protein intake. He argued against what he called "capsule eating," or taking vitamins.

He also called for regular fasting, or, as he called it, "rest-fasting." A fast lasting anywhere from five to thirty days could, he said, restore health at the cellular level, allowing the body to restore its natural practices, recover its vitality, and rejuvenate itself. He wrote,

"A great change in cell life and structure takes place during a fast and it is well to continue the fast until this change is complete and nothing but healthy tissue remains. In this way a new body emerges from the process. It is thin, but ready to be re-built upon normal lines."

Shelton noted that many athletes already understood the benefits of fasting and habitually fasted for a period of days as part of their training. At the same time, he stressed that for most people, fasting should be undertaken carefully – ideally at a Hygienic facility. Just as people should not eat "haphazardly," they also should not fast haphazardly.

A body treated well – treated hygienically – will preserve its own health, Shelton argued. That's the kernel of his beliefs, and it's also the reason that he was so virulently opposed to mainstream medicine. He railed against what medical drugs, calling them "poison." But beyond that, he urged his followers to look at health, and disease, in a whole new way:

"Hygienists are not engaged in curing disease. Indeed, we hold that ill efforts to cure disease are based upon false notions of the essential nature of disease. Disease is a process of purification and reparation. It is not an enemy of the vital powers but a struggle of the vital powers themselves in self-defense. We of the Hygienic school do not regard the diseases which are said to kill so many every- year as of themselves, dangerous; we hold that the great mortality seen in these diseases is due to suppressive and combative treatment. Disease is not a thing to be removed, expelled, subdued, broken up, destroyed, conquered, or cured or killed. It is not a thing, but an action; not an entity, but a process; not an enemy at war with the living organism, but a remedial effort; not a substance to be opposed, but an action to be cooperated with."

Looked at correctly, Shelton believed, disease is not an enemy. It is an opportunity to improve one's own relationship to our bodies. It is an opportunity to reconnect with our native vitality and to come into deeper connection with the restorative forces of nature. At a time when more and more of us are living anxious lives, increasingly disconnected from the physical and natural world, Shelton's writings seem more relevant than ever.

— Jessica Wheatley

THE DEVELOPMENT OF DISEASE

After disease has reached a more or less advanced stage, or after the patient is dead the condition of the body in such states has been thoroughly studied. Diagnosis is the art of discovering effects, and these cannot be discovered until after they have reached a certain stage—until after they have advanced far enough to produce a physical sign. In the *descending pathological transit* a certain series of changes must necessarily occur before the damage becomes great enough to manifest as signs and symptoms, and these changes require time. When a pathological condition becomes manifest so that a diagnosis, right or wrong, may be made, this is not its beginning. Indeed, its beginning may be, and often is years prior to this. Its development is invariably slow, gradual, insidious, causing little or no disturbance to the body and no visible sign of its presence.

What of these initial stages? What of the stages which precede the production of a physical sign? Cause is here at work for weeks, months or years and the pathological condition is gradually developing. The individual imagines he is healthy and refuses to believe that his mode of living is harming him. His physician may examine him and tell him that he is alright, that all of his organs are sound, and yet, the condition that is later to manifest itself by physical signs and symptoms is developing. From this class of "healthy" individuals gradually emerges the many cases of advanced organic disease. These "pre-clinical" stages are the most important stages in the development of such conditions as cancer, insanity, paralysis, paresis, locomotor ataxia, Bright's disease, diabetes, diseases of the heart and arteries, cirrhosis of the liver or kidneys, etc., etc. If these "pre-clinical" stages are prevented the advanced stages will not develop.

The "Modern" methods of dealing with such conditions are faulty in that they consider an individual to be healthy, however evil his mode of living, if no physical signs of "disease" are to be found. The causes that produce these signs are wholly ignored; perhaps unknown to medical men. Indeed there is still "more truth than poetry" in Trail's observation made in relation to the various schools of medicine of the past:—

"One source of error, however, pervaded all their observations, as it does postmortem investigations at this day. It is this: Structural appearances after death denote the effects of disease; and these morbid changes were and are often mistaken for or confounded with the causes of disease."—*Hydropathic Encyclopedia*, Vol. I, p. 31.

"Medical Science" still goes to the dead and dying in its search for cause. Critical studies and examinations of end-results are the means employed in searching for causes.

"Functional derangements," says Dr. Tilden, "are of the same nature and from the same universal cause that ends in all organic so-called diseases. All so-called diseases are, from beginning to end, the same evolutionary process. All symptom complexes— diseases—from their initiation to their ending, are effects, and the most intense study of any phase or stage of their progress will not throw any light on the cause."—*Toxemia Explained*.

At a necropsy, the chest of a young man who had died of tuberculosis of the lungs was opened revealing an ugly abscess of one of the lobes of the lungs. "There," said one of the physicians present, "I don't want to look any further for the cause of death."

But he was looking at the end, not at the beginning of the young man's trouble. How come the abscess there? How come the liver diseased? How and why do congestions, inflammations, etc., develop? Such conditions as was revealed in opening this young man's chest do not come into existence full-blown, any more than trees or flowers do so. Diseases never come butt-end first and Jennings truly said: "The ground is first broken at the surface, and there is a regular gradation from the summit level of physical soundness to the stagnant fenny region of disorder. It takes a great while and an amazing amount of opposing, noxious influences to reduce a healthy vigorous human system to a diseased state, according to the common acceptation of that term."—*Philosophy of Human Life*, p. 100.

There is no organic disease without previous functional disease; and there can be no functional disease except under a deficiency of functional power. Post-mortem examinations and physical examinations by the physician reveal effects, results, end products, not causes. Let us trace the development of pathology from its initial beginnings to its final endings.

In tracing this development, let us first get a general view of the processes of life. The nutritive functions of the body may be roughly divided in two classes, namely:—

I. Those by which food is prepared for use by the body, and distributed to all parts of the body, and finally, used by its cells and organs.

II. Those by which waste and injurious matter is broken down, prepared for excretion and carried to the excreting organs and, finally, eliminated.

By the joint operation of these two general functions, the body is built up and sustained, on the one hand, and kept clean and pure on the other. Its perfection in size, symmetry and form, depends upon the integrity and efficient activity—granted a proper supply of building material—of these two functions.

Under the most natural and healthful activities of the vital organism there is necessarily a constant wear and impair of organic substance, necessitating a constant process of repair to prevent the rapid wearing out of the organic machinery. While, therefore, the general nutritive functions are efficiently and vigorously sustained, no sooner does any substance in the body become unfit for further use than it is caught up by the lymph vessels and hurried along to the blood and to its final expulsion from the body, while its loss is immediately made good by fresh material brought there by the lymph.

By these two processes, a sound body, after attaining maturity, if the laws and conditions of life and health are complied with, will retain for a long period, its identity of size, form, weight and complexion, while, at the same time, undergoing constant change, its tissues and organs being daily and hourly in process of renewal.

The powers of the various organs of the body may be appropriately classified as *fundamental* and *special*. The processes of building a machine must always be distinguished from the processes of the machine after it is built. The processes by which the body is built, and the processes by which the body or any of its organs works after it is ready for function are different. The evolution of a kidney is one kind of a process. The production of urine by the completed kidney is another kind of process. Every organ and part of the body may, therefore, be said to possess two powers—namely: (1) Its power of self-repair and self-maintenance, which is its *fundamental* power; and, (2) Its functioning power, that is its power to work, which is its *special* power. These powers are inherent in the organs or in their cells, although in the body they are governed and controlled by the nervous system and while this is true of both powers, it is especially true of the special power.

The *fundamental* power maintains the organ in repair and in readiness for work when supplied with motive power by the nerves. It heals its wounds, removes its worn out cells and replaces these with new ones and repairs its damaged structure. This work is largely dependent upon the blood and lymph for its success.

Jennings called this power the *recuperative function*, and pointed out that so long as there is sufficient power to maintain repairs no organic defects will or can develop in an organ for as rapidly as it sustains wear and tear this is repaired and structural soundness is maintained. It is only after the body has been abused and weakened so that its various parts are no longer fully capable of recuperating and repairing themselves as rapidly as they sustain wear and tear that the various organs of the body begin to take on change.

Let us for convenience break up the development of disease into three distinct stages or steps, keeping in mind, at the same time, however, that there are no distinct lines of demarcation between these stages. They are all of a piece and each shades gradually, imperceptibly into the other. In doing this we have:—

First: *Declension of power*: No portion of the living organism ever takes on disordered action, except where it suffers great violence, until its energies have been reduced to a point below that necessary to sustain it in normal function. The vital properties were made to act just as they do under the circumstances in which they act, and they possess neither disposition nor power to act in any other way. The highest possible good of the organism in general, and of its several organs in particular is the end always before the forces of life and toward this end they aim as steadily and unerringly as the needle to the pole. When all parts are well supplied with power, there is GOOD HEALTH, general and local. When there is a deficiency of functioning power, that is, less power than is required to sustain a healthy functional standard, the health of the part or parts is IMPAIRED, and impaired to the extent of its lack of power.

By virtue of the *law of life*, each organ of the body has a specific and distinct function to perform, which it must perform, or attempt to perform, while it has the power to act. The vigor and efficiency of any function, and the perfection of its work, is proportioned to the ability of the organ to labor—a due supply of appropriate material being understood.

As an example, the liver must secrete bile, and supply this just when, in the exact quantity and precise quality required, if there is power enough at the command of the vital economy to effect this. If there is not sufficient power to enable the liver to supply perfect bile as required, the liver must meet its obligations in this particular according to the power it possesses and not according to the power it does not have.

Second: *Impairment and derangement of function, functional disease*: When the energies of an organ or group of organs have been reduced to a point below that essential to the maintenance of healthy function, its functions are impaired or deranged. In a sound state of the body, when all the parts are sufficiently supplied with power, there may be a large temporary diminution of the power of one or more organs of the body, without any derangement of function, but when the general stock of energy is reduced to a supply barely adequate for ordinary use, any reduction below that level must be followed by derangement When such a condition exists and the body is subjected to circumstances that require more energy to maintain its functions at the standard-level of comfortable health, than is required under the usual conditions of life then impairment of function must follow. Sudden and great changes in weather, exposure, fatigue, overeating, excitement, grief, shock, prostrate the greatly enervated, not the vigorous and strong.

Every organ and part of an organ is liable to functional impairment as a result of a reduction of its sustaining energy. The manifestations, or symptoms, which announce the defective state of the part or parts, will depend on the organ or parts of the organ affected, and the extent of the affection.

A change in the substance or structure of an organ, can only be reached through functional impairment and derangement and this can only take place through a pinching scantiness of functional power. There is, in all violations of the laws of life, an actual loss of power, but, as Jennings said, "We have no vitometer by which to graduate this defect; and it is only when power is reduced so low that action falters, or structure changes that we can begin to measure the damaged condition of the body; and from this point the symptoms become our guide, and our only guide to a knowledge of the quality or kind, seat and extent of disease—in the *common* use of the term."

Although the action of pathoferic substances is primarily and directly, upon the substances of the organs of the body, yet the injurious effect would be discovered first—if we had means of measuring the vitality of its parts—in a reduction of power. For even in a tolerable sound and vigorous body, there is power in reserve, over and above what is necessary for ordinary purposes. This capital stock of energy, over and above the usual expenditures, is held in store for an emergency, and while, therefore the draft upon this reserve is increased by every assault, the supply necessary for the work of maintaining functional action and structural integrity will be furnished till the reserve is exhausted. After this, if the demand for power to sustain functional soundness exceeds the income, the organ or organs must falter in their functions, and here commences FUNCTIONAL DISEASE.

Dr. Tilden admirably traces the development of functional diseases as follows:— "The stomach is the most abused organ of the body. Almost immediately after birth the child is often enervated from fondling and overfeeding. Meddlesome midwifery, called modem medical science, enervates both mother and child, rendering the mother's milk, if there is any milk at all, unfit as food. Very soon after birth, symptoms of indigestion appear in the child, and as often in the mother, which automatically starts a cinema of infant-feeding and care that competes in exquisite torture with the inventions of the fiends of hell. Here is laid the foundation for the universal gastrointestinal catarrh that extends on and on, involving more or less all the mucous membranes of the body, becoming the father of all diseases *peculiar* to children—all the diseases recognized as catarrhal: colds, croup, tonsilitis, and others of the respiratory organs, all of which are reflex irritations of gastro-intestinal catarrh. And, as the skin is the mucous membrane without the body, the extension of the catarrh at times reaches the surface of the body, manifesting itself in one form or another of the exanthematous or eruptive gastro-intestinal catarrhal diseases, including smallpox. Respiratory diseases and eruptive diseases are interchangeable. (It was learned in the chapter on *Crises* that the suppression of the exanthemata most often results in respiratory and other mucous membrane complications and sequelae. Author's note).

"This brings us to the relationship of pneumonia and smallpox—the former an extension of gastro-intestinal catarrh to the lungs, and the latter an extension of gastrointestinal catarrh to the surface of the body. Both these types of disease vary from a light, almost insignificant derangement to a malignancy that is fatal in almost every case. The cause of the great difference in severity, from almost nil to fatal malignancy, is the state of the body—it is a question of the degree of Toxemia. In pronounced enervation and Toxemia, with gastro-intestinal putrescence from an excessive intake of animal protein, infection from absorption of the intestinal decomposition, added to the existing Toxemia, often builds a fatal malady."—*Philosophy of Health*, Aug. 1924.

Third: *Structural impairment or change— organic disease.* Every part of the body is susceptible of change or impairment of its structure and substance, to a greater or less extent. This results from functional derangement which, in turn, results from enervation. When the fundamental or recuperative power of an organ is unable to repair itself as rapidly as it wears out or is damaged, a change in structure ensues. Every day happenings evidence the fact that wounds and broken bones heal without difficulty even under unfavorable external circumstances and that there are cases where neither cuts, bruises, or broken bones will heal under very favorable external circumstances. When power is low and the blood exceedingly foul the ability of an organ to repair and renew itself is greatly impaired. In toxic states of the body there is more or less destruction of the functioning cells of the body, and these, due to the ease with which they are destroyed by the toxins, instead of being replaced by others of their own kind are replaced by a functionless substitute of connective tissue or "scar tissue," which is better able to live under the circumstances. The damaged section of the organ is repaired by this tissue—the only tissue that may be used for repair under the circumstances. Thus, even cirrhosis or the hardening of an organ is a defensive measure, one designed to prolong life as long as possible. The forces of life always work for the preservation of life and when they cannot do as well as they would, they do as well as they may.

In functional derangements there is ordinarily more or less change of structure; but as this is only temporary, and the parts are soon restored to the natural state, it is not regarded as organic disease. It is only when functional derangement has persisted long enough that these changes have become extensive and permanent, that the condition is regarded as organic disease. Thus it will be seen that functional and structural diseases shade insensibly into each other. Structural disease does not always end in death, nor does functional derangement always result in organic change.

First, then, there must be exhaustion of power below a certain standard before there can be impairment or derangement of function. Impaired function must be impaired still more and prolonged before structural derangement can take place.

Want of power, then, the most vital kind of power, is the immediate cause of impaired, or what is called morbid or diseased action, for nothing constitutes good health, the highest degree of vigor, but a full and overflowing state of the vital treasury in every department of life. And not only should the fountain of supply abound and superabound, with vital energy, but every tissue and organ, and all the fluids and secretions of the body should & sound, and pure. Unfortunately, in the present state of mankind, there are no perfect constitutions, and but few that can be rightly clued as sound or good. One or more organs of the body are weak and faulty. They are more easily brought into a state of disease than the stronger more perfect ones, and take an organic change more readily when through oft repeated, protracted and aggravated violations of physical law, nature is unable, uninterruptedly, for any length of time, to maintain a nice balance between waste and repair.

The loss of power that must precede the development of disease is due to waste of power largely occasioned by the use of irritants and excitants—stimulants. Hence the egregious folly of the habitual employment of stimulants or tonics of various kinds, until the vital economy is forced to hang out its distress signals, and then employing the same means in larger amounts, or others of similar character and greater power, to remedy the damages of the habitual over-stimulation.

When over-stimulation has lashed an organ into impotency and organic change is taking place nature calls loudly for a let-up in activities. If this is granted the work of cure proceeds. The most rigid economy is exercised in the expenditure of power. Reinforcements are called in as far as can be done without incurring greater peril in some other organ, and every favoring circumstance is employed to avert, if possible, the ruin of a vital organ. Depleted energies hold out for a time, then lag behind for a brief period, then as if having gathered fresh strength, they rush forward in a greater effort and regain what they had previously lost. But if no change is made in the mode of living, and cause is not corrected, and as the treatment employed produces more enervation and more damage to the body the forces of life are worn down. The unequal contest finally balances against feeble vitality. The organs of elimination "fail to remove the cumulative mass of useless matter," as Jennings puts it, and wastes are no longer adequately repaired. Another stage in the pathological descent is reached— ORGANIC DISEASE.

The development of organic disease is never sudden and never without repeated warnings. Their earliest stages are purely functional and, as previously pointed out are evanescent. If causes are corrected they never become organic.

Let us assume that an infant begins life with semi-perfect health. He is fed too much and too often. He is bundled up too much, denied fresh air and sunshine, handled too much and subjected to too much noise. Colic develops. The baby cries. He is fed and drugged. Colds, constipation, punctuated with frequent diarrhea, skin rashes, tonsilitis, etc., develop. The stomach and bowels become sensitive. Indigestion becomes a "habit." Gastritis, bowel diseases, sore throat, the exanthemata, or erruptive diseases develop as crises. Chronic catarrh develops.

A sensitive stomach, enlarged tonsils, adenoids, impaired bowel action, glandular swellings and perhaps richets and other troubles follow the child through the next few years of white bread, potatoes, cakes, candies, pie, cereals with sugar, milk, eggs, meat, and repeated drugging. Frequent crises develop and these are palliated or suppressed. Puberty arrives and this may carry them by sheer force of developmental power through adolescence with but a part of their childhood troubles or with none of them.

After adulthood is reached there comes indigestion, nausea, vomiting, gastritis, sleeplessness, headaches and pains in various parts of the body.

In women painful menstruation develops, if indeed they have not had this from the first. They become morbid, and perhaps more or less hysterical.

The excesses and dissipations of this period from twenty to thirty-five, coupled with imprudent eating and frequent drugging—cathartics, headache remedies, bicarbonate of soda, etc.—and operations soon lay a secure foundation for chronic disease. Anemia, gastric ulcer, visceroptosis, chronic rheumatism, tuberculosis, etc. develop. At first these symptoms are only functional and periodic but as the causes are continued and intensified the affected organs undergo structural changes. From their functional beginnings in infancy to their organic endings in middle life these so-called diseases represent a continuous development out of ever increasing causes. Every chronic disease is of slow development and cannot exist without previous systemic impairment. Each toxemic crisis is palliated by drugs or treatment that produce greater enervation and build a greater toleration for toxemia. Chronic diseases are the legitimate outcomes of palliated acute troubles. Dr. Tilden well pictures the gradual evolution of disease in these words:

"When the organism is enervated from the thousand-and-one influences incident to life, and intoxication has brought on such a state of metabolism that the organism is overwhelmed by waste—excretory products—it is then that inherited diathesis takes on activity. If the diathesis is tubercular, gouty, neurotic, or of any of the special organs of the body, it is in keeping with the laws of health and life for the affection peculiar to the diathesis to spring up. If the causes are not removed, the affection will remain functional for a time; then organic change will take place. It is then that affections became diseases; it is then that irritation and an inflammation from indigestion become ulceration of the bowels or stomach, and the ulcer perforates, and death ensues from peritonitis caused by the perforation. The peritonitis was caused by the perforation; perforation was caused by ulceration; ulceration was caused by inflammation; inflammation (catarrh) was caused by irritation; irritation was caused by indigestion; indigestion was caused by fermentation; fermentation was caused by enervation; and enervation was caused by the thousand-and-one influences which build or destroy the body and mind of men, depending on whether they are wisely or unwisely applied."—*Impaired Health*, Vol. 1, p. 258.

Despite the evident looseness in the use of terms, the above description of the development of disease conditions is excellent. Each step is built on or out of the preceding one as a result of the continued operation and intensification of the same cause or causes. It were rank folly to regard disease in any other light.

Catarrh is a hypersecretion of the mucous membranes made necessary by plethora or a full habit—an overcrowded state of the blood-vessels—and by irritants and excitants. It is a conservative measure—a natural means of relieving the blood pressure and the engorged state of the mucous membranes. When this conservative measure is worked overtime there results a gradual impairment of function followed by inflammation of the mucous membrane. This passes into ulceration.

The poisons produced by carbohydrate fermentation give rise to the simple forms of inflammation such as are seen in colds, catarrh, etc. If no more food is eaten than can be fitted for use by the body, secretions and excretions are closely enough balanced to maintain health. If the body is abused by excess of all kinds, by overclothing, living in overheated, poorly ventilated houses and by overeating, then passing from a hot room into the cold outdoors, or from a warm bed into a cold room will set up enough irritation of the exposed mucous membranes to bring on congestion—a cold, catarrh, hay fever, bronchitis, laryngitis, pharyngitis, etc.

Where enervation is pronounced, due to mental and physical habits that use up nerve force to excess, secretion and excretion are impaired. They fall below the level demanded by health. There is a consequent increase in the amount of waste matter circulating in the blood. If, as is usual, the accustomed amount of food is eaten, or if some unusual drain upon the nervous energies is sustained, digestion will not be perfect. Secretion will not be adequate to the work of digesting all the food eaten and there will be some left over which will fall to the bacteria, that are always present in the digestive tract, to be broken down. Fermentation and putrefaction will occur. A catarrhal inflammation of the stomach, intestine, or other part of the body will be set up. The catarrhal condition becomes general and forms the foundation for the development of many affections of the body.

Where the catarrh develops in the stomach and intestine, as in gastritis, it may easily spread to the common bile duct and from this to the gall-bladder and other bile ducts, even passing on into the liver itself.

Gastritis is the same condition in the stomach as a cold is in the nose and throat. Back of it are the same causes that produce a cold. Chronic catarrh of the stomach and intestine is the same thing as chronic catarrh of the nose and throat. Back of these conditions are the same causes. An acute catarrhal inflammation of the common bile-duct or of the gall-bladder is simply a "cold" in these parts; while a chronic catarrhal condition of these organs, is the same condition as a chronic catarrh of the nose and throat. Back of each of these conditions are the same causes.

The excessive use of sugar, cakes, pies, bread, cereals, milk, etc., are the chief causes of catarrh. Of course, in all cases enervation must check elimination, else out-go will be made to equal income and health will be maintained.

That person who conserves his nervous energies, who does not indulge in excesses and dissipations, who eats sensibly and moderately, who secures plenty of rest and sleep, who takes daily physical exercise, and who secures an abundance of fresh air and sunshine, will not be troubled with catarrh or any other disease.

A cold does not produce other diseases as is popularly taught and generally believed. The constitutional derangement, enervation, toxemia and intestinal indigestion which brought on the crisis (cold), also builds the other "diseases," even the organic "diseases." Not one cold but many colds and other crises develop over the long period of time during which organic disease is developing.

Nephritis is a disease of infancy and youth. It occurs largely from the ages of one to ten, following usually upon the suppression of scarletina or other febrile disease, and from twenty to thirty when the dissipations of young men reach their maximum. Degeneration of the kidneys belongs to middle age and beyond, when the "habits of life begin to tell."

A man goes along in average health until he reaches the age of forty. There are occasional headaches, colds, perhaps gastritis, and constipation for which he uses laxatives, but he feels well most of the time, is "never sick," has a good appetite, is never forced to be absent from his work because of illness, and he therefore considers himself in good health. Then at forty from one cause or another he has an examination made and discovers that he is suffering with diabetes which is considerably advanced. Nature's repeated warnings had gone unheeded and now he is paying the penalty. These pre-clinical symptoms—discomforts and mild functional disturbances—Orthopathy regards as marking the commencement of the second division of the descending pathological transition: the first manifestation of waning vitality. This is the answer to the question once put to Dr. Jennings: "My wife has a *fever*, what has that to do with *living*?"

A lady became sick enough to call in a doctor. Her trouble was palliated in the usual way. Trouble after trouble developed while others remained. For years she suffered with intestinal catarrh when ulceration developed. During this time she was operated on eight times. Gall-stones and probably the gall-bladder were removed, the appendix and coccix bone were each removed. Three operations were performed on the rectum and two sinus operations were performed. Finally cancer of the intestine developed.

Her physicians regarded each of her affections as distinct diseases, of local origin, and the removal of the affected organ was supposed to cure the disease. That they represented local manifestations of a general or systemic condition, that they all stemmed from the same basic cause, were mere steps or stages in the progressive degeneration of the woman's body, did not enter into their considerations. That there was any connection between intestinal catarrh and the gall-stones, appendicitis or ulcer, or that intestinal catarrh and sinusitis were the same condition in two locations did not enter into their philosophy.

Chronic disease may begin in the liver or pancreas or kidney and develop gradually and insiduously until the affected organ is beyond repair before the owner of the organ becomes aware that there is anything wrong with him. He may consider himself to be in good health. He practices certain destructive habits for years. He is apparently in good health. His friends indulge in the same habits. His doctor and nurse do likewise. Nothing arouses his suspicions that he is not in good condition. He does not even suspect that his habits are not all right. Then, at forty he begins to fail rapidly. Perhaps there is a sudden development of uremia. An examination shows him to be in the advanced stages of chronic Bright's disease with his kidneys beyond repair. He suddenly finds that all the time he was boasting that "nothing hurts me, I do as I like," "I can eat anything," "I always enjoy three square meals a day," "tobacco never hurts me," "alcohol won't harm one if he takes it in moderation," and imagining himself in good health, he was really standing with one foot in the grave, and the other on a banana peel.

Such a condition does not develop suddenly. It is the result of causes that operate in the daily life of the individual. These causes are found almost wholly in the voluntary habits of the person. Back of the first observable symptoms of decline were many small aches and pains, colds and periods of not feeling very well. One crisis after another arose and subsided, but these were considered unimportant and their causes ignored.

Back of these signs of developing chronic disease is another period in which the disease is developing but not making itself felt. During this stage no method of examination now known can detect the developing disease, although a knowledge of cause will enable one, by analyzing the person's mode of life, to declare that some forms of disease is developing.

Back of the clinical signs, back of the pre-clinical signs, when the disease is developing but not manifesting itself in any manner, there are its causes. Disease is a development. It no more comes into existence full-blown than flowers or trees do, the germ theory to the contrary notwithstanding. Its beginnings are small, imperceptible; its development slow, gradual, insidious. The disease begins where cause begins and persists where cause persists. The clinical phenomena of disease, the pre-clinical phenomena of disease and the unobservable phenomena of disease are not separate and distinct stages of disease. They are all of a piece and all shade off imperceptibly into each other. They are all evolutions out of the same causes and are continuous because their causes are continuous.

Men who study disease, that is its symptoms and results, and who look upon these as causes or as entities are led into many rather serious blunders. They regard a given affection as being due to the failure of some organ and treat the organ.

When eating habits are such as to crowd the liver functions—impair its functions of urea formation, detoxification, and preparing sugar for use or for elimination— kidney troubles arise as a consequence. But the failure of the liver's functions is not the cause of the kidney trouble. It is one of the causes, but is secondary to the primary cause, overeating or imprudent eating. Rational treatment would correct the eating instead of treating the liver or kidneys.

The same mistake is made with regard to constipation. There is hardly a disease in the nosology which this common complaint is not accused of causing. By some it is even considered to be the chief cause of cancer.

It is not correct to say constipation causes this or that disease, headache, rheumatism, cancer, etc. It is rather nearer the truth to say that the causes of constipation are also the causes of these "diseases." We must get away from the prevalent manner of viewing constipation as a cause and learn to see it as an effect. It may be objected that when the constipation is cured the headache ceases or that no cancer will develop. It would be equally as correct to say that when the headache is cured the constipation is cured also. They are concomitant effects of the same cause or causes and not one the cause of the other. When the causes of constipation are removed the causes of cancer are also removed.

Those who regard constipation as the cause of their ills attempt to cure their ills by the use of purgatives, laxatives, enemas, wheat bran, etc., while those who regard constipation as part of their ills, a mere symptom, get rid of all their troubles by correcting and removing the common cause of all of them. Thus it will be seen that in practice it makes all the difference in the world which of these views we adopt.

Under the first view the very means employed to cure the constipation invariably make it worse. They irritate, depress, enervate and further inhibit function, and if continued long enough cause a complete cessation of function.

Two "diseases" (tonsilitis and metritis, for instance) existing together or successively are concomitant or successive effects of a common cause, an extension of effects of one cause, and not cause and effect of one another. It is the state of the blood that goes to both the affected organs that causes the disease in each and not the inflammation in one organ that causes the inflammation in the other. The recurrent development of crises in an organ or tissue is due to the continued operation of the original producing causes. The subsequent or concomitant development of a crisis in another organ in a remote part of the body is due to the extension of these same causes.

Obviously, if the causes which result in some bodily disorder or local inflammation, or which lead to the formation of some growth or to the hardening of some tissue, are permitted to continue acting after the inflammation or disorder has subsided, or after the growth has been removed, either a recurrence of the disease or the development of some "other" and, what is most likely, more extensive disease or a worse growth must develop. How often do we see people suffer from repeatedly recurring attacks" of some disorder! How often does this condition continue to extend and grow worse and "other" diseases develop! The individual who has sore throat or bronchitis or gallstones or headache may and usually does get another and another "attack" of the same trouble, because, as soon as one crisis is over he begins to build another. A simple ovarian tumor is removed. A few months or a few years later it is followed by another or by the formation of a cancer about the stump of the simple tumor. This indicates that the operation of the same causes that produced the first tumor, when not corrected, produce a second and that the primary causes of simple tumors and of malignant or cancerous tumors are the same.

The blood circulates throughout the whole system, and, if it is abnormal in any respect every part of the body must suffer more or less as a result. It is not accidental which part or parts of the body are affected most. If the blood is normal the parts of the body will be well nourished and properly cleansed, and, in the absence of some more or less accidental local causes, which may momentarily disturb some part, will be able to maintain their structural and functional integrity. Should they be subjected to local irritation, this will soon be remedied, by the circulation of healthy blood in the part, and very soon all traces of the former irritation will be gone. The irritation will be in proportion to the magnitude and duration of the exciting cause, the resistance of the part being great because of its soundness and because of the wholesomeness of its blood supply, so that the suffering caused by the irritant is comparatively slight.

But let the blood be foul—toxic—that is, loaded with waste and re-fuse and the effects of such an irritant will be much greater and more slowly recovered from. It will occasion greater suffering. Take, for instance, a wound of the leg which heals readily and with little suffer-ing in those of sound health and pure blood, but which, where health is impaired and the blood is foul heals slowly, or not at all, and occasions great suffering. The suffering in such a case would be "proportionate to the magnitude of the injury and inversely as the healthiness of the blood, or proportionately to its unhealthiness." A. Rabagliati, M.A., M.D., F.R.C.S., Edin, a reformed British medical man declares:

"Most local ailments are only local expressions of general states. The specialist is by implication here relegated to his proper place, and is informed, if he has wit enough to read the lesson presented to him, that it is not sufficient to remove an ovarian tumor, e. g., and that if nothing is said at the same time or subsequently as to the causes which induced it, a positive damage may be done to the woman, who may, therefore, while considering herself cured, proceed to manufacture one on the other side, or may find herself in a few years suffering from cancer in the stump of the previous one. Or the child who has tonsils removed, and adenoids cleared away, may and certainly will subsequently suffer from colds, bronchitis, broncho-pneumonia, and the like, and bye and bye probably from rheumatism or rheumatic fever, etc., unless at the same time or subsequently to the operation, his mother is advised to treat him differently from the way in which she treated him before. For, if she does not, a worse thing may happen to him in the future, and so the operation which was intended to benefit may eventuate in damage and not in good. Evidently the same causes which enlarged the tonsils and caused the adenoid growths, on the soft palate and nose will, if they are allowed to go on, tend to make the child ill again either in the same or in some other way. Or the middle-aged woman, who has a chronic discharge from her nose, may get it stopped, indeed, by having her nose cauterised by a platinum wire made white hot by the electric current, only to find herself in a few months suffering from a cancer of the breast, which, being in turn removed, eventuates in cancer of the liver, for which there is no relief. These illustrations are, I may say, by no means imaginary, but are drawn from experience of cases in practice."—*Air, Food and Exercises*, pp. 129-130.

Local affections or local inflammations are far more serious as be-ing marks of the general condition of the blood, than they are as being mere local affections. If then, a sick person presents a number of "local diseases" they are not to be considered as independent or idiopathic diseases, nor yet as symptomatic diseases, one derived from the other, but as concomitant or successive effects of a common cause. Thus when a man presents arthritis in one or more joints, valvular heart disease, or myocarditis, and tonsilitis, the first named local affections are not to be considered as having been caused by the tonsilitis, and as curable by removal of the tonsils, but these affections and the tonsilitis are to be regarded as being due to a common fundamental cause and all, alike, curable by correcting or removing this common cause. Patients often develop endocarditis first, then arthritis and then tonsilitis last. It is a bit hard to make tonsilitis responsible for these other two conditions when they develop in advance of the tonsilitis. It is just as logical in such a case to say that the endocarditis or arthritis caused the tonsilitis as, in other cases, to hold tonsilitis responsible for these other conditions. The only tenable view is that the three conditions have a common origin, even if this does knock the idea of specific diseases due to specific causes into a cocked hat and support our contention for a unitary cause, and the unity of disease. That disease, from first to last is all of a piece was declared by Jennings in the following words:

"There is no propriety in the common mode of computing physical defection—that part of it that obtains the appelation of disease. Whatever name is given to physical degeneracy should be made to include the whole of it, first, second, and third stages. It is all a damaged state, alike needing recruit and replenishment. The gradation in the line of degeneracy, from the elevated point of perfect structural and vital soundness to the commencement of the second stage where functional disturbance begins, must always be a lengthy one; for the distance between the two points is immense, and cannot be traversed by noxious agencies in one or two generations. It would be impossible by any mode or degree of abuse to reduce a sound body to a condition in which fevers, pleurisies, bilious affections, colds, etc., could be manifested. The vital economy might be broken up and destroyed by a great variety of violent methods, and the different parts of the body might be reduced by long-continued and excessive exercise to a tired weary point; but the individual organs could not be made to take on the ordinary forms of impaired health. There are men in this degenerate age—men, too, who fall far short of physical perfection—who go on to a very advanced period of life under a constant strain upon their vital machinery from noxious agencies and practices: who never have colds, coughs, fevers, or any serious illness—'are never sick a day in their lives.' They are proof against 'the pestilence that walketh in darkness, and the destruction that wasteth at noon day.' These men have vital force enough within call in every department of their systems to guard against injuries and repair damages without the necessity of making a palpable demonstration of unsoundness.

"These cases, however, instead of constituting the universal rule, as ought to be the case, are but slight exceptions among the great bulk of mankind that are near the lower border of the first grade of degeneracy, verging toward the second grade, constantly liable, from a low state of vital powers, to be hurried into it."—*Tree of Life*, pp. 117-18.

Dr. Page agrees with this statement and expresses it as follows:

"The fact is that there is a process of degeneration going on throughout the entire structure of the man, even to the last tissue, and the symptoms are all indicative of this; and this is more or less strictly true of all disorders. The naming and classifying of 'disease' is calculated to mystify and mislead; sickness is the proper term for describing them all: self-abuse, in the broadest sense of the word, is the cause of them; and obedience to law, the only means of prevention or cure."—*The Natural Cure*, p. 131.

Page, who regarded diphtheria as "only a phase of albuminuria," quotes one Dr. Grasmuck as saying "Another peculiarity of the scourage is its fondness for children of a certain condition—the fat, sleek, soft, tender, 'well-fed' children so generally admired—such children can offer but slight resistance to this disease; being in fact, chronically diseased, they are predisposed to 'attacks' of all kinds; and, living to adult age, furnish the greater proportion of cases of tuberculous disease. On the other hand, I do not know of a single instance where the disease proved fatal to—rarely attacking— a child of the genus 'Street Arab'—children who spend most of their time out of doors, are thinly clad, sleep in cold rooms, have a spare diet, and who have no one to pamper them unwisely."

Inflammation of the respiratory organs—pleurisy, pneumonia, bronchitis and MEMBRANOUS CROUP—often accompany Bright's disease. Whether these conditions and diphtheria are phases of albuminuria and whether or not we accord any place to germs in their production we must recognize those prior causes which prepare the body for the development of these troubles. And we must cease repeating the old error about fat, sleek, ruddy, well-fed children being healthy. Jennings said:

"Let it be remembered that no variety nor degree of 'rosy cheek' is an indication of health, but contrawise, a mark of a very serious constitutional defect"—*Medical Reform*.

Upon this same point Graham declared:

"There is another thing concerning which a general error of opinion prevails. It is a common notion that a florid countenance, when not produced by intoxicating liquors, is a sure sign of good health, and that a pale complexion is an invariable indication of poor health. It is true that there is a kind of sallow, sickly paleness which is a pretty sure sign that the functions of the system are not all healthfully performed; but it is far from being true that a ruddy countenance is always the index of good health; and still farther from being true that it is always the index of that health which is most compatible with long life. 'Too much ruddiness in youth,' says Hufeland, 'is seldom a sign of longevity.' As a general fact, at all periods of life, it indicates that state of the system in which, either from disease or from intensity, the vital expenditure is too rapid for permanent health and for longevity. The clear complexion in which the red and white are so delicately blended, as to produce a soft flesh-color, varying from a deeper to a paler hue according as the individual is more or less accustomed to active exercise in the open air, or to confinement and sedentary and studious habits, is by far the best index of that kind of health and of that temperament which are most favorable to continued health and length of days."—*Science of Human Life*, p. 495.

And lastly, Page says of this common error:

"This symptom (red cheeks) popularly regarded as a sign of health, is simply evidence of plethora when it is habitually observed in robust individuals, young or old, and denotes a predisposition to febrile disease. *Congestion of the cheeks* is, of course, not dangerous, in itself considered, but it is no more a sign of health than is congestion in the bowels, lungs or kidneys: It is a note of warning and should be promptly heeded. The plethoric, or full-blooded, robust subject should be more abstemious in diet—taking less food as a whole, perhaps, or adopting a less stimulating and non-irritating diet. The frail, delicate, or anemic patient's flushed cheeks are not apt to be misinterpreted." —*How to Feed the Baby*, p. 136.

Hale looking men with a moderately full and florid countenance live fast and die prematurely. The florid countenance is due to a moderate and habitual distension and congestion of the capillaries of the face. It is an evidence of plethora or the full habit, of over-stimulation or what Graham called *vital intensity*. How frequently do we meet with fresh, hale looking men who go on to forty or sixty years of age, apparently in good health and then who sink rapidly and die!

A total abandonment of all irritants, other things remaining the same, is always followed by the establishment of a better and more permanent state of health accompanied by a corresponding abolition of the facial congestion.

If the stimulant user possesses a sound, vigorous constitution, and no other overpowering causes intervene, "very good health" will be enjoyed for years, with occasional slight interruptions such as colds, pains, bowel disturbances, etc., but the constant action of irritating matter upon sensitive organs will at length call for reparation.

Where this condition is due to overeating, it will be necessary to eat more moderately and perhaps to revolutionize the diet. For, it should be remembered that considerable quantities of meat, eggs, bread, condiments, spices, etc., will produce such a countenance until the health is so impaired that the blood is impoverished and one takes on the appearance of anemia. A knowledge of the conditions of health will enable us to avoid disease.

The study of the pathological changes which occur in an organ in chronic disease, let us say in the kidneys in Bright's disease, is all very well for the technician, although as Dr. Page observes, "If *too much time* is devoted to it, and to the *relation of drugs* thereto, by an individual, he may be, probably will be, the very least fitted to advise an inquirer who desires to know what he can do to be saved from disease and the supposed necessity of taking medicine."

Now "From a practical standpoint" as Page says, "when a man's sickness is attended with a certain set of symptoms, as albumen in the urine, final suppression of the urine and uremic poisoning—occasioned by a peculiar degeneration of the kidneys, we care nothing about the kind of change taking place in the kidney, but rather ask what kind of change in our habits will keep this, and all other organs of the body in a healthy condition." To put this more simply, the study of the conditions of health is of far greater importance than is the study of pathology after this has developed from a failure to comply with the conditions of health.

Medical men usually begin at the finish to diagnose a disease. After the patient is dead they hold a post-mortem and their findings are handed out as a diagnosis. They find a cancer, a fibroid tumor, an abscess and these are given as the cause of death. But these things are effects. They are the results of causes that are not discoverable at the necropsy, causes that have ceased. They see the finished product, not its initial beginnings and hence, are not able to learn anything that is of value in preventing such developments.

Tumors and cancers have long been a serious problem in medical circles. Little is yet known in these circles of their causes and development and this we feel is due largely to the fact that they continue to regard them as specific entities requiring specific causes for their production and fail to recognize their oneness with the other pathological states of the body and their origin out of the pathoferic causes which produce these other pathological states.

They are regarded chiefly as a disease of middle life and old age. They are seldom found in children and young people and there must be a good and sound reason for this.

It is probably correct to say that children do not suffer from cancer for the reason that their habits have not had time to produce it. A few cases do develop in children, who must be predisposed to its development, and the number who develop the disease increases as age increases, due no doubt to the fact that the causes which produce the disease continue to accumulate and grow in power as age advances. The causes operating to produce cancer take time to act and it is for this reason that cancer becomes more common as age increases.

In childhood and early life irritation in the body is accompanied by intolerance. The young organism vigorously resists the causes of irritation and throws them off. This gives rise to the fevers, inflammations, sudden and fierce, and frequently of short duration, so characteristic of childhood.

As age advances and the tissues harden they cease to offer such violent resistance to irritation, but tolerate it, so that the diseases of middle life and beyond are not so fierce as in childhood and youth. The ever increasing cause begins to weigh down and depress the powers of the body The ordinary powers of resistance to toxins and irritants and the usual means of disposing of surplus food are impaired and the body is forced to defend itself and dispose of its surplus food by some more or less unusual means. New growths of all kinds are composed of cells and in order to grow it is necessary that more food material be brought to them than is necessary for the sustenance of the normal tissue of the part. Long continued local over-nutrition due to irritation or circulatory obstruction would seem to be necessary for the immediate production of a neoplasm.

There are many kinds of tumors but these are broadly grouped as (1) connective tissue tumors, (2) epithelial tissue tumors, and (3) mixed tissue tumors, that is, tumors composed of mixtures of various tissues. Wood defines a tumor as "a more or less circumscribed collection of cells arising wholly independently of the rest of the body, in general growing progressively, and serving no useful purpose in the organism." He admits that this definition is entirely descriptive and adds "as we do not know the cause or causes of tumors it is impossible to define these structures more accurately." In dealing with their classification he makes a similar statement, saying: "Inasmuch as we do not know the cause of tumors, it is impossible to make a strictly scientific classification of them. It is, therefore, most convenient to use a purely morphological basis for classification, drawn from the microscopic appearance of the tumors and the tissues from which they originate. Cysts are included with tumors because of their genetic relationship to new growths rather than to any other pathological condition."

We object to two features of this definition—we do not see how it can be maintained that tumors grow independently of the body; and, we are certain that they do serve a useful purpose in the organism. It will not be denied that those portions of a cyst, or at least some cysts, which are genetically related to neoplasms serve a very definite and eminently useful purpose. A cyst which forms around a foreign body, a parasite for example, is definitely useful and protective.

From our standpoint a "strictly scientific classification" of tumors is not necessary, for they represent the same condition, or the same process in different tissues and are the results of the same causes acting on the different tissue? Tumors may develop in any organ or any tissue of any organ in the body and they derive their names from these organs and tissues. Thus, myoma is the name given to a tumor of muscle tissue; endothelioma the name applied to a tumor developing in the endothelium of some of the body's cavities; osteoma a bone tumor, etc., etc. These names relate to tissues, organs and locations—the differences in these tumors are those derived from the differences that exist in the tissues in which they originate. When the variation from the normal type of tissue in which the tumor originates passes beyond a certain more or less indifinite line the tumor becomes malignant. This represents merely another stage or step in the pathological evolution and not the addition of some new element. It is the result of the continued action of the original producing causes.

From these considerations it is evident that tumors are a unit just as inflammation is a unit. Furthermore, they do not represent distinct and specific "diseases," but are merely links in a long chain of causes and effects which extend backward in the life of the individual to infancy, perhaps, beyond.

A female infant suffers with colic, frequent colds, constipation, frequent diarrhea and "hives" or frequent skin rashes of one form or another. As she grows older there are colds, sore throats, enlarged tonsils, "children's diseases," frequent spells of nausea and vomiting, etc. With the arrival of puberty there occurs painful and irregular menstruation, accompanied with headaches, styes on the eyelids, pains in the back, nervousness, loss of appetite and other symptoms. Later indigestion develops and this is palliated, as were all the preceding troubles, with no attention given to cause. The palliative measures afford her immediate relief, but remotely aggravate the indigestion they were used to relieve. She now has frequent recurrences of some one or more ailments like headache, or neuralgia, or colds, or "bilious attacks," or rheumatism, or she is constantly fatigued, and finally becomes chronically ill. Finally at about the age of thirty or thirty-five she is discovered to be carrying a large ovarian tumor. Now it seems hardly correct to single out the tumor from among all the train of symptoms and ills which this woman has suffered, beginning in infancy and lasting throughout her whole life, and decide that its development has no connection with these prior troubles, that it is a distinct and specific disease depending on some specific cause and wholly unrelated to the causes which have been producing her ills from infancy onward.

Multiple tumors, that is two or more tumors in the same individual supply us with an interesting confirmation of our theory of the unity of tumors and the unity of cause. These may develop in any tissue in the body or in several different tissues in which case they resemble the tissues from which they arise.

Irritation—mechanical, chemical, thermal, actinic, etc.—is among the undoubted causes of cancer. But irritation alone is not sufficient to produce tumors or cancer. Tumors of the skin on the face are frequently multiple. So also are tumors arising from x-ray burns or from irritation from coal tar. In such cases a unitary cause is recognized. When there is long continued chronic irritation over a large area the tumors are usually multiple. Unity of cause is here again recognized.

But it is argued that the presence of a carcinoma of the uterus and of a carcinoma of the stomach must be based on different irritants. When tumors are found to exist in some portion of the intestinal tract and also in one or both ovaries, the intestinal tumor is regarded as primary and the ovarian tumor as secondary, being derived from the primary one by *metastasis*. Metastasis is the name applied to the theory that particles of tumors break off or are detached from the parent body and are carried by the blood or lymph to other parts of the body where they attach themselves and begin the development of another tumor.

All of this, I regard as a fanciful hypothesis supported only by the artificial production of tumors—that is the occasional production of a tumor in an animal by inoculation with particles of tumor from another animal. Such experiments can throw no light on the causes of tumors for the very simple reason that no human being ever develops cancer by any such method.

Wood records a case of epithelioma of the lip "which remained fairly localized and was successfully removed by operation with no recurrence at the end of a year." However, by this time there had developed a very large carcinoma of the thyroid, all the lymph-nodes of the neck being involved along with the surrounding tissue. The patient died. At autopsy no traces of the epithelioma of the lip were found in regional lymph nodes and adjoining parts of the face but numerous small carcinomata were present. Both carcinoma and sarcoma may develop in the same individual concomitantly or successively, and some instances are recorded in which both types of these tumors have existed together in the same organ. These are especially found in the uterus.

Now all of these phenomena we regard as arising out of the same primary cause. The development of a tumor in one organ or tissue is due to the same cause that produces a tumor in another organ or tissue. Instead of multiple tumors, when these exist in different organs, being due to metastasis, we regard them as originating out of the same primary cause. They are not primary and secondary to each other, but concomitant or successive developments from a common basis. Wood records a case of development of carcinoma of the uterus ten years after the removal of a carcinoma of the breast and says that "Metastatic connection between the tumors could be ruled out."

If the irritants that help to produce tumors are to be regarded as always acting from without, and never from within, then it may be right to say that carcinoma of the stomach and carcinoma of the uterus arise from different irritants. But this assumption is by no means necessary and besides, the irritant is a secondary and not the primary cause of the tumor. I do not doubt that sexual self-abuse, eroticism, excessive intercourse and most, if not all contraceptive measures tend to the production of tumors of the female genital organs.

Carcinoma and sarcoma are the two chief forms of cancer and represent special forms of hyperplasia of epithelial and connective tissue. Epithelioma or carcinoma is cancer of the epithelial tissues; sarcoma, as distinguished from carcinoma is cancer of the connective tissues. Sarcoma and carcinoma are doubtless both due to the same causes acting on different tissues. These causes occasion an overgrowth of these structures, two or more cells appearing where before was only one. Once this process has started it continues, under the continued operation of the producing causes, "constantly spreading, ulcerating or fungating by advance and recession. The advance, however, preponderating through necessity until ultimately its break down results in death."

Hypertrophy, hardening and hyperplasia are due to over-nutrition and to irritation. These processes pushed beyond what we may term *physiological limits*, give rise to ulceration and cancer. They begin as conservative or defensive measures and they continue as such. There is no doubt, in the writer's mind, that except for the development of those conditions known as tumors and cancers, the causes which necessitated them would destroy life much sooner than they do. In other words the development of tumors and cancers prolongs life. I have no doubt that their development is in the highest degree orthopathic; that they develop only when there is an urgent necessity for just such developments.

No laws are violated in their development I am equally confident that if their causes are corrected before they have grown too large, nature will tear down these conservative measures, for they, like all conservative measures, are only intended as temporary measures.

H. W. S. Wright, M.S., F.R.C.S. says: "There can be no doubt that in nearly all cases there is what may be called a precancerous stage. It is moreover a long standing chronic condition which, as a rule, gives rise to very little inconvenience on the part of the patient. After this *precancerous* stage there appears what may be called *early cancer*, often indistinguishable to the naked eye from the original precancerous lesion, but giving rise to great suspicion in the eyes of the initiated on account of its hardness, and tendency to be fixed."

In a handbook of *Essential Facts about Cancer*, prepared for the medical profession by a special committee of the *American Society for the Control of Cancer*, I find the following words, 'A factor which, during the last ten years, has proved to be of great importance in the causation of cancer, is chronic irritation. As the various theories of the parasitic origin of cancer have been disproved, chronic irritation has been found increasingly to be an important factor in the incidence of cancer in one region or another." This is the opening paragraph of a chapter devoted to "precancerous conditions," and among these conditions are listed and discussed such things as fissures, chronic ulcerations and indurations (hardenings), irritation from gall-stones, erosions and lacerations of the cervix of the womb, chronic cystitis, old burns, scars, the effects of x-rays and radium, etc., while "many tumors which are essentially benign in character" are said to be "capable of malignant transformation, especially in the later years of life."

Cancer at the start is not cancer. It may be a gastric ulcer, or an x-ray or radium burn, or a fistulous rectum, or a torn cervix, or a hardened fundus or a chronically inflammed ovary. What produces this change? Why does last year's ulcer, for instance, become this year's cancer? Obviously, it is an evolution out of the prior condition and due to the same causes perhaps intensified, that produced the prior condition.

Premature ageing, or sclerosis of the tissues and blood-vessels may exist to such an extent that they can offer but little resistance to the causes of ulceration. This is undoubtedly a factor when essentially benign tumors undergo "malignant transformation in the later years of life." Other causes may intervene to cut off oxygen and nourishment so that putrefaction sets in followed by systemic infection. Or, drainage may be cut off forcing absorption and the development of blood-poisoning—cancerous cachexia. Poisoning by cancer is a form of sepsis slowly generated and liberated in the system.

Whatever the cause of the development of a cancer out of a pre-cancerous condition, an ulcer, induration, fistula, benign tumor, etc., it is only another step in the *downward pathological transit*, a condition that would not have developed had the precancerous condition not first developed, and so closely related is it to the preceding condition that it is not possible to tell just where the pre-cancerous condition ends and cancer begins. The folly of attempting to prevent cancer by the surgical removal of the pre-cancerous state should be obvious when it is realized that the causes of the condition lie back of it and cannot be removed by the knife. Indeed the knife frequently occasions the rapid development of a cancer.

The tissues of some people are more susceptible to the development of tumors than are the tissues of other people, and some tissues in the same person are more susceptible to its development than others. Dr. Bulkley thinks there is a *cancer-diathesis* just as there is a *tubercular diathesis, a gouty diathesis*, etc. When a chronic irritant is applied to those tissues of an individual which are "susceptible" to cancer such a condition is much more apt to develop than when applied to other tissues or to the same tissues of another individual. But this state of susceptibility is not, beyond a weakened state of the tissues, due to any inherent predisposition to tumor development. It is undoubtedly due to toxemia of a virulent character.

Irritation causes an extra amount of blood to be sent to the point of irritation causing congestion and inflammation. In all cases of inflammation there is rapid cell proliferation and an overgrowth of tissue. But, where the system is sound and the blood pure the irritation is soon overcome, the inflammation subsides and the excess of tissue is broken down and carted away. Where the blood is foul its accumulation at a point of irritation increases the irritation and, unless the condition of the blood is changed, tends to perpetuate the low-grade inflammation that is thus set up in old people. Those tissues which are most resistant to the toxins and are not killed by these multiply as in all inflammations and as the irritation is continuous, the inflammation is continuous and growth is continuous. Irritation, inflammation, ulceration, induration and cancer is the order of development.

Tilden thus traces the development of a fibroid tumor:—

"A young woman develops intestinal indigestion from imprudent eating. The catching-cold habit, with catarrh of the mucous membranes, follows. Soon there is developed intestinal putrefaction, which being absorbed, causes infection. The pelvic lymphatics become involved. As there is more or less congestion of the mucous membrane lining the uterus and its neck, this condition is made more pronounced each month because of menstruation and the toxins being absorbed in the bowels. The uterine engorgement causes longer and more profuse menstruation; painful menstruation begins, growing more pronounced month by month. Pain forces the calling of a physician, who on examination finds a flexed womb. The flexion is caused by a thickening of one side of the womb, which forces a flexion to the opposite side. The more thickening the more obstruction to the circulation and the more bent is the neck of the womb; and the more bent is the neck, the more the canal is obstructed to the menstrual flow.

"As the womb is flexed more and more, the circulation is more and more interfered with. The flexed side fails to receive the proper amount of nourishment, and the thickened side receives all that the uterine and other vessels can bring; but the return vessels fail to carry back the full amount, and, as a result, hypertrophy takes place— the parts are overstimulated. Nature undertakes to organize the surplus; and she does —and we call it a fibroid tumor. These growths grow rapidly or slowly according to the amount of obstruction.

"A growth may fill the pelvis and abdomen in five years; and again in some other women it may require twenty years to develop a tumor the size of an orange.

"Injuries at childbirth often become the first cause of tumor, next to putrefactive infection from intestinal indigestion.

"Another cause: A catarrhal inflammation locates at an old placental site, as a result of toxemia. Thickening and induration follow, impeding the efferent circulation. The more growth, the more pressure and obstruction, until the new growth—fibroid tumor—is large enough to become a cause of its own growth, by impeding the circulation through its weight and pressure.

"This work of overgrowth is pushed along rapidly by overeating, which means over-nourishing; the surplus being organized into tumor.

"Overeating and improper eating often cause gas distention of the bowels. The pressure from gas crowds and misplaces the womb. From such misplacements enough obstruction to uterine circulation may take place to cause hypertrophic enlargement, which is fibroid enlargement;

"Constipation may cause enough pressure on the womb to start imperfect circulation, and later fibroid growth.

"Wherever there is impeded circulation, new growth must take place; and that means tumor. The kind of tumor will depend on the character of the tissues involved.

"Add to these causes sclerosis, and malignant diseases may follow. That is, the benign tumors may become malignant."—*Impaired Health.* Vol. 1, pp. 255-6-7.

A tumor is not only composed of cells of the same kind as those composing the tissue from which it is derived, but these cells are frequently functioning tissue. Carcinoma of the thyroid often secretes the specific thyroid material, a tumor of the breast is apt to contain structures which remind us of the secreting glands of the mamma; a uterine tumor is likely to contain involuntary muscle fiber, carcinoma of the bowel often contains glandular structures which closely resemble the normal structures of the intestine, and which secrete mucous.

However, the tumor as a whole does not resemble perfectly normal tissue. In a fibroma, for instance, its connective tissue cells are absolutely identical with those of the tissue in which the tumor is situated, but the general structure is usually more or less cellular than the normal connective tissue. Blood vessels have thin walls, or in dense tumors, are almost entirely absent over considerable areas. The lymph channels are defective, while the nervous structures present have no relationship with the tumor. These latter merely pass through the tumor to the normal structures which they innervate. In tumors in cartilaginous structures (chondioma), the cartilage is not so regular in structure as in normal cartilage. In tumor of the bone the bone cells and lamellae are not so systematically arranged as in normal bone.

From this it should be evident that these structures will break down more easily than normal tissue once their nutrition is cut off or their drainage is impaired. They would undergo decomposition and sepsis would develop.

The degenerative changes which occur in the various types of tumors, benign and "malignant," do not differ from the alterations which occur in normal tissues when the blood supply is diminished or ulceration and cachexia have developed. Due to the imperfect character of their capillary circulation, and to the usually insufficient blood supply, and to thrombosis which results usually from pressure or stasis, tumors are more liable to hemorrhage and subsequent degeneration than is normal tissue. Hemorrhage, various types of degeneration, often beginning with fatty degeneration of its cells which may progress to calcifications or even bone formation, and leading ultimately to necrosis or gangrene result from pushing the tumor beyond the boundary of safety. And this is done by the continued operation of the producing causes. If these causes are corrected in time these changes will not occur and the tumor will be reduced somewhat or, perhaps, be completely absorbed.

A lady, age fifty-six, came to the writer in the early part of 1926, suffering with a variety of ailments, digestive disturbances, headaches, high-blood pressure, constipation, pains in the back, excessive weight (she was over forty pounds overweight), and multiple myoma of the uterus. Thirty days on no food but water followed by two months on a diet of fruits and green vegetables, resulted in the loss of all of these affections including forty pounds of weight and the myomata. At this writing, fifteen months from the time the case was dismissed there has been no recurrence of any of her troubles, nor of the myomata. She was saved from a hysterectomy which was urged upon her by four different physicians, and since she is living an entirely different life to what she formerly led, I am confident she will never experience a recurrence of the tumors, unless she returns to the former mode of living.

However, I believe we are correct in general when we say that, when the body has reached such a low state of deterioration and degeneracy that it develops cancer it is next to impossible for regeneration to take place to an extent necessary for the restoration of health. In a large majority of those cases operated on recurrence occurs in from six months to four years, while in the few where recurrence fails to occur there is grave doubt about them ever having been cancer.

I have seen numerous small tumor-like developments quickly disappear under a hygienic regimen and I have seen many enlarged and hardened lymph glands, which had been diagnosed as tumors, soften and become normal in size, often doing this very quickly. I have saved many women from needless operations on their breasts for supposed cancers.

There are five considerations which we would leave with the reader:

1. Those pathological phenomena called tumors or cancers are merely links in a syndrome of causes and effects operating in the life of the individual and are genetically connected with the pathology which precedes them.

2. They constitute a unit, one form of tumor with another form, and also with preceding pathological developments.

3. They are conservative and protective measures and serve to prolong rather than to destroy life.

4. These conditions while undoubtedly easily eradicated in their early stages, in most cases, by remedial hygiene, are not curable by any means after they have advanced beyond a certain stage.

5. They are easily preventable, the prevention depending upon a hygienic mode of living.

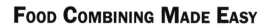

FOOD COMBINING MADE EASY

Dedication

To the millions of truthseekers everywhere, who are desirous of knowing more about healthful living, in the hope that it will serve them in preserving and restoring their health and the health of the members of their families, this book is affectionately dedicated by

—The Author

INTRODUCTION

I have been requested hundreds of times to provide my readers with a small book on food combining. The demand has grown with the years as more and more people have come to realize the importance of properly combined meals. In offering this little book to the public I hope to meet the requirements of the layman whose knowledge of the technical side of the matter is limited. I have written the book in plain language and have provided sufficient technical data to make the subject clear to the average reader.

As the book has been prepared for the general reader and not for the vegetarian only, the menus contained herein include meals for the mixed-diet eater as well as meals for the vegetarian. This has not been done as a matter of compromise, nor yet as a tacit desertion of vegetarianism, but as a means of meeting the requirements of all classes of readers.

From medical sources, as well as from the camp-followers of medicine in the other schools of so-called healing, and the dietetic camp-followers of allopathy, certain objections are made to the practice of avoiding certain food combinations and eating others. These objections are all based on the assumption that the human stomach is equipped to easily and efficiently digest any and all possible combinations of foods that may be introduced into it. Very little special attention will be devoted to meeting these objections, as the facts presented in this little book constitute sufficient reply to the objections. Should the reader desire further refutation of these objections, they may be had in my larger work, *Orthotrophy*, which is Vol. II of *The Hygienic System*.

More than thirty-one years spent in feeding and caring for the young and the old, the well and the sick, male and female, rich and poor, educated and ignorant, nearly twenty-five years of this spent in institutional practice, the balance in office practice, certainly entitle me to speak with some degree of authority on this subject. I have spent more than forty years in the study of dietetics, and I have directed the care and feeding of many thousands of people. I submit to the intelligent reader the thought that such an experience better qualifies me to speak upon the subject that forms the text of this little book than an equal time devoted to drugging the sick. Few medical men make a study of dietetics and still fewer of them make any extensive use of it in their care of their patients. Their usual advice to their patients is to "eat whatever agrees with you."

Dr. Shelton's Health School has been in existence here in San Antonio since July 10, 1928. During this time patients have come to it from all over the United States and Canada and from many parts of the world. Mexico, Argentina, Nicaragua, Costa Rica, Brazil, Venezuela, Cuba, Hawaii, China, New Zealand, Australia, England, Ireland, South Africa, Alaska, and other parts of the world have contributed patients to the Health School. The marvelous results we have obtained and are obtaining in our care of all classes of sickness, even in thousands of cases that had been declared to be "incurable," attest the value of the methods and measures employed in the Health School.

It is not asserted in this book that any program of diet, nor any program of food combining, will cure disease. I do not believe in cures. I assert and am ready to prove, that in all cases of sickness, where organic damage is not too great for vital redemption, when cause is removed the forces and processes of life, working with the normal materials of life, will restore health and integrity. Food is but one of the normal materials of life.

As an indispensable basis of the work of the *Hygienist,* we must endeavor to secure to the patient the full benefit of all the *hygienic* means, in their entire plenitude, for only thus can the patient be given a fair chance of recovery. The intelligent reader should have no difficulty in understanding that *Hygienic* care is the only rational and radical care that has ever been administered to the sick in any age of the world at any place. The time must come when all forms of disease will be "treated" on the broad and infallible basis of *Hygienic* principles. When true principles are discovered, they are found to apply, not to one or two diseases only, nor to but one class of diseases, but to all diseases whatsoever. The same fundamental principles will apply throughout the whole catalogue of diseases. Even in those cases where surgery can be of value, *Hygienic* care should always be employed as the groundwork for the surgery.

The Health School is ideally located in the sunny southwest where summers are mild, the days fanned with the southerly winds of the gulf, the nights cool, winters are short and mild, with sunbathing all winter, where the soil is the finest and there is a year-round profusion of the finest fruits and vegetables in the world. These natural advantages, added to our vast experience in handling all forms of disease, enable us to offer the health seeker care and direction that are not available elsewhere.

At the Health School we employ all of the materials and influences that have a normal relation to life—air, water, food, sunshine, rest, sleep, exercise, cleanliness, emotional adjustment, etc. Physiological rest—fasting—also occupies a prominent place in our system of care. But first and foremost in our care of the sick is the removal of the causes that are responsible for the disease. Trying to cure disease without removing its cause is like trying to sober up a drunk man while he continues to drink. We would not attempt a thing so foolish.

Our patients are fed correctly combined meals. These things are set down here that the reader may know that the rules for food combining given in succeeding pages are not merely theoretical considerations, but that they have been fully tried and tested in the crucible of wide experience.

Why give attention to the combinations of foods eaten? Why not combine our foods indiscriminately and eat haphazardly? Why give thought and attention to such matters? Do animals follow rules of food combining?

The answers to these questions are simple. Let us start with the last question. Animals eat very simply and do very little combining. Certainly the meat eating animal consumes no carbohydrates with his proteins. He does not take acids with his proteins. The deer grazing in the forest combines his foods very little. The squirrel, eating nuts, is likely to eat his fill of nuts and take no other food with these. Birds have been observed to eat insects at one time of day, seeds at another. No animal in a state of nature has the great variety of different foods spread before it at a meal that civilized man has. Primitive man had no such great variety of foods at a meal. He, too, ate simply, as do the animals.

As will be seen later, the digestive enzymes of the human digestive tract have certain well defined limitations and when we eat in such a manner as to over ride these limitations, we run into digestive troubles. Proper food combining is merely a sane way of respecting our enzymic limitations. We combine our foods properly and do not eat haphazardly and indiscriminately, because, by so doing, we assure better and more efficient digestion of our foods.

We derive no value from foods that are not digested. To eat and have the food spoil in the digestive tract is to waste the food. It is worse than this, as the spoiling of foods results in the production of poisons which are injurious. Proper food combining, therefore, not only assures better nutrition, as a consequence of better digestion of our foods, but it provides for a protection against poisoning.

An amazing number of food allergies clear up completely when supposedly allergic individuals learn to eat their foods in digestible combinations. What they suffer from is not allergy, as this is at present understood, but indigestion. Allergy is a term applied to protein poisoning. Indigestion results in putrefactive poisoning, which is also a form of protein poisoning. Normal digestion delivers nutrients, not poisons to the bloodstream. Fully digested proteins are not poisonous substances.

With knowledge based on wide experience, then, I offer this little book to the intelligent reader, in the hope that he will make full use of its information to the end that he may enjoy better health and a longer and more abundant life. To the doubter I say only: Give it a trial and convince yourself. It has truly been said that condemnation without investigation is a bar to all knowledge. Do not cut yourself off from further knowledge and from better health by condemning, without a fair test, the simple rules that are presented in this little book.

CHAPTER I

Foodstuffs Classified

Food is that material which can be incorporated into and become a part of the cells and fluids of the body. Non-useful materials, such as drugs, are all poisonous. To be a true food the substance eaten must not contain useless or harmful ingredients. For example, tobacco, which is a plant, contains proteins, carbohydrates, minerals, vitamins and water. As such, it should be a food. But, in addition to these materials, it also contains considerable quantities of poisons, one of these, one of the most virulent poisons known to science. Tobacco, therefore, is not a food.

Foodstuffs as we get them from the garden and orchard or from the food store, or in the raw state, are composed of water and a few organic compounds known as proteins, carbohydrates (sugars, starches, pentosans), fats (oils), mineral salts and vitamins. They commonly possess more or less of non-usable or indigestible matter-waste.

Foods as we get them from the garden and orchard or purchase them from the food store are the raw materials of nutrition. They vary widely in character and quality, hence, for convenience, are classified according to their composition and sources of origin. The following classifications of foods will guide the reader in his combinations.

PROTEINS

Protein foods are those that contain a high percentage of protein in their makeup. Chief among these are the following:

Nuts (most)	All flesh foods (except fat)
All cereals	Cheese
Dry beans	Olives
Dry peas	Avocados
Soy beans	Milk (low protein)
Peanuts	

The carbohydrates are the starches and sugars. I have broken these up into three distinct groups in the following classification— starches, sugars and syrups, and sweet fruits.

STARCHES

All cereals
Dry beans (except Soy Beans)
Dry peas
Potatoes (all kinds)
Chestnuts
Peanuts
Hubbard Squash
Banana Squash
Pumpkin
Caladium root
Jerusalem Artichokes

MILDLY STARCHY
Cauliflower
Beets
Carrots
Rutabaga
Salsify

SYRUPS AND SUGARS
Brown sugar
White sugar
Milk sugar
Maple syrup
Cane Syrup
Honey

SWEET FRUITS
Banana
Date
Fig
Raisin
Tompson & Muscat Grape
Prune
Sun-dried Pear
Persimmon

FATS

The fats are all fats and oils, as follow:

Olive oil
Soy Oil
Sunflower Seed Oil
Sesame Oil
Corn Oil

Butter
Cream
Nut oils
Butter substitutes
Pecans
Avocados

Most nuts
Fat meats
Lard
Cotton seed oil
Tallow

ACID FRUITS

Most of the acids eaten as foods are acid fruits. Chief among these are

Orange
Grapefruit
Pineapple
Pomegranate

Tomato
Lemon
Lime
Sour Apple

Sour Grape
Sour Peach
Sour Plum

SUB-ACID FRUITS

The sub-acid fruits are as follow:

Fresh fig	Sweet Peach	Huckleberry
Pear	Sweet apple	Mango
Sweet Cherry	Apricot	Mangosteen
Papaya	Sweet Plum	Cherimoya

NON-STARCHY AND GREEN VEGETABLES

Into this classification fall all succulent vegetables without regard for their color, whether green, red, yellow, or white, etc. Chief among these are:

Lettuce	Cow-slip	Parsley
Celery	Chinese cabbage	Rhubarb
Endive (French)	Chive	Water cress
Chicory	Chicory	Onions
Cabbage	Mustard	Scallions
Cauliflower	Dock (sour)	Leeks
Broccoli	Turnip	Garlic
Brussel Sprouts	Kale	Zuccini
Collards	Mulliein	Escarole
Spinach	Rape	Cardoon
Dandelion	Green corn	Bamboo Sprouts
Beet tops (greens)	Egg-plant	Broccoli-de-Rappe
Turnip tops	Green beans	Summer squash
(greens)	Cucumber	Asparagus
Chard	Kohl-rabi	Radish
Okra	Sorrel	Sweet pepper

MELONS

The melons are as follow:

Water melon	Casaba	Crenshaw melon
Musk melon	Cantaloupe	Christmas melon
Honey dew	Pie melon	Persian Melon
Honey Balls	Banana melon	Nutmeg Melon

CHAPTER II

Digestion of Foods

Foodstuffs, as we eat them constitute the raw materials of nutrition. As proteins, carbohydrates and fats, they are not usable by the body. They must first undergo a disintegrating, refining and standardizing process (more properly a series of processes) to which the term digestion has been given. Although this process of digestion is partly mechanical, as in the chewing, swallowing and "churning" of food, the physiology of digestion is very largely a study of the chemical changes foods undergo in their passage through the alimentary canal. For our present purposes, we need give but little attention to intestinal digestion, but will concentrate upon mouth and stomach digestion.

The changes through which foods go in the processes of digestion are effected by a group of agencies known as enzymes or unorganized ferments. Due to the fact that the conditions under which these enzymes can act are sharply defined, it becomes necessary to give heed to the simple rules of correct food combining that have been carefully worked out on a basis of the chemistry of digestion. Long and patient effort on the part of many physiologists in many parts of the world have brought to light a host of facts concerning enzymic limitations, but, unfortunately, these same physiologists have attempted to slur over their importance and to supply us with fictional reasons why we should continue to eat and drink in the conventionally haphazard manner. They have rejected every effort to make a practical application of the great fund of vital knowledge their painstaking labors have provided. Not so the *Natural Hygienists*. We seek to base our rules of life upon the principles of biology and physiology.

Let us briefly consider *enzymes* in general before we go on to a study of the enzymes of the mouth and stomach. An *enzyme* may be appropriately defined as a physiological *catalyst*. In the study of chemistry it was soon found that many substances that do not normally combine when brought into contact with each other, may be made to do so by a third substance when it is brought into contact with them. This third substance does not in any way enter into the combination, or share in the reaction, its mere presence seems to bring about the combination and reaction. Such a substance or agent is called a *catalyst*, the process is called *catalsis*.

Plants and animals manufacture soluble catalytic substances, colloidal in nature and but little resistant to heat, which they employ in the many processes of splitting up of compounds and the making of new ones within themselves. To these substances the term *enzyme* has been applied. Many *enzymes* are known, all of them, apparently, of protein character. The only ones that need interest us here are those involved in the digestion of foodstuffs. These are involved in the reduction of complex food substances to simpler compounds that are acceptible to the bloodstream and usable by the cells of the body in the production of new cell-substance.

As the action of enzymes in the digestion of foodstuffs closely resembles fermentation, these substances were formerly referred to as ferments. Fermentation, however, is accomplished by organized ferments—bacteria. The products of fermentation are not identical with the products of enzymic disintegration of foodstuffs and are not suitable as nutritive materials. Rather, they are poisonous. Putrefaction, also the result of bacterial action, also gives rise to poisons, some of them very virulent, rather than to nutritive materials.

Each enzyme is specific in its action. This is to say, it acts only upon one class of food substance. The enzymes that act upon carbohydrates do not and cannot act upon proteins nor upon salts nor fats. They are even more specific than this would indicate. For example, in the digestion of closely related substances, such as the disaccharides (complex sugars), the enzyme that acts upon maltose is not capable of acting upon lactose. Each sugar seems to require its own specific enzyme. The physiologist, Howell, tells us that there is no clear proof that any single enzyme can produce more than one kind of ferment action.

This specific action of enzymes is of importance, as there are various stages in the digestion of foodstuffs, each stage requiring the action of a different enzyme, and the various enzymes being capable of performing their work only if the preceding work has been properly performed by the enzymes that also precede. If *pepsin*, for example, has not converted proteins into peptones, the enzymes that convert peptones into amino acids will not be able to act upon the proteins.

The substance upon which an enzyme acts is called a *substrate*. Thus starch is the substrate of *ptyalin*. Dr. N. Phillip Norman, Instructor in gastro-enterology, New York Polyclinic Medical School and Hospital, New York City, says: "In studying the action of different enzymes, one is struck by Emil Fischer's statement that there must be a special key to each lock. The ferment being the lock and its substrate the key, and if the key does not fit exactly in the lock, no reaction is possible. In view of this fact is it not logical to believe the admixture of different types of carbohydrates and fats and proteins in the same meal to be distinctly injurious to the digestive cells? If, since it is true that similar, but not identical locks are produced by the same type of cells, it is logical to believe that this admixture taxes the physiological functions of these cells to their limit." Fischer, who was a renowned physiologist, suggested that the specificity of the various enzymes is related to the structure of substances acted upon. Each enzyme is apparently adapted to or fitted to a certain definite structure.

Digestion commences in the mouth. All foods are broken up into smaller particles by the process of chewing, and they are thoroughly saturated with saliva. Of the chemical part of digestion, only starch digestion begins in the mouth. The saliva of the mouth, which is normally an alkaline fluid, contains an enzyme called *ptyalin,* which acts upon starch, breaking this down into maltose, a complex sugar, which is further acted upon in the intestine by *maltase* and converted into the simple sugar *dextrose.* The action of ptyalin upon starch is preparatory, as maltase cannot act upon starch. *Amylase,* the starch-splitting enzyme of the pancreatic secretion, is said to act upon starch much as does *ptyalin,* so that starch that escapes digestion in the mouth and stomach may be split into maltose and achroodextrine, providing, of course, that it has not undergone fermentation before it reaches the intestine.

Ptyalin is destroyed by a mild acid and also by a strong alkaline reaction. It can act only in an alkaline medium and this must not be strongly alkaline. It is this limitation of the enzyme that renders important the manner in which we mix our starches, for if they are mixed with foods that are acid or that provide for an acid secretion in the stomach, the action of the *ptyalin* is brought to an end. We will learn more of this later.

Stomach, or gastric juice ranges all the way from nearly neutral in reaction to strongly acid, depending upon the character of the food eaten. It contains three enzymes—pepsin, which acts upon proteins; lipase, which has slight action upon fats; and rennen, which coagulates milk. The only one of these enzymes that needs concern us here is pepsin. Pepsin is capable of initiating digestion in all kinds of proteins. This is important, as it seems to be the only enzyme with such power. Different protein splitting enzymes act upon the different stages of protein digestion. It is possible that none of them can act upon protein in stages preceding the stage for which they are specifically adapted. For example, *erepsin,* found in the intestinal juice and in the pancreatic juice, does not act upon complex proteins, but only upon peptids and polypeptids, reducing these to amino-acids. Without the prior action of pepsin in reducing the proteins to peptids, the erepsin would not act upon the protein food. Pepsin acts only in an acid medium and is destroyed by an alkali. Low temperature, as when iced drinks are taken, retards and even suspends the action of pepsin. Alcohol precipitates this enzyme.

Just as the sight, odor or thought of food may occasion a flow of saliva, a "watering of the mouth," so these same factors may cause a flow of gastric juice, that is a "watering of the stomach." The taste of food, however, is most important in occasioning a flow of saliva. The physiologist, Carlson, failed in repeated efforts to occasion a flow of gastric juice by having his subjects chew on different substances, or by irritating the nerve-endings in the mouth by substances other than those directly related to food. In other words, there is no secretory action when the substances taken into the mouth cannot be digested. There is selective action on the part of the body and, as will be seen later, there are different kinds of action for different kinds of foods.

In his experiments in studying the "conditioned reflex," Pavlov noted that it is not necessary to take the food into the mouth in order to occasion a flow of gastric juice. The mere teasing of a dog with savory food will serve. He found that even the noises or some other action associated with feeding time, will occasion a flow of secretion.

It is necessary that we devote a few paragraphs to a brief study of the body's ability to adapt its secretions to the different kinds of foodstuffs that are consumed. Later, we will discuss the limitations of this power. McLeod's *Physiology in Modern Medicine* says: "The observations of Pavlov on the responses of gastric pouches of dogs to meat, bread, and milk have been widely quoted. They are interesting because they constitute evidence that the operation of the gastric secretory mechanism is not without some power of adaptation to the materials to be digested."

This adaptation is made possible by reason of the fact that the gastric secretions are the products of about five million microscopic glands embedded in the walls of the stomach, various of which secrete different parts of the gastric juice. The varying amounts and proportions of the various elements that enter into the composition of the gastric juice give a juice of varying characters and adapted to the digestion of different kinds of foodstuffs. Thus the juice may be almost neutral in reaction, it may be weakly acid or strongly acid. There may be more or less pepsin according to need. There is also the factor of timing. The character of the juice may be very different at one stage of digestion from what it is at another, as the varying requirements of a food are met.

A similar adaptation of saliva to different foods and digestive requirements is seen to occur. For example weak acids occasion a copious flow of saliva, while weak alkalies occasion no salivary secretion. Disagreeable and noxious substances also occasion salivary secretion, in this instance, to flush away the offending material. It is noted by physiologists that with at least two different types of glands in the mouth able to function, a considerable range of variation is possible with reference to the character of the mixed secretion finally discharged.

An excellent example of this ability of the body to modify and adapt its secretions to the varying needs of various kinds of foods is supplied us by the dog. Feed him flesh and there is a secretion of thick viscous saliva, chiefly from the submaxilary gland. Feed him dried and pulverized flesh and a very copious and watery secretion will be poured out upon it, coming from the parotid gland. The mucous secretion poured out upon flesh serves to lubricate the bolus of food and thus facilitate swallowing. The thin, watery secretion, on the other hand, poured out upon the dry powder, washes the powder from the mouth. Thus, it is seen that the kind of juice poured out is determined by the purpose it must serve.

As was previously noted, ptyalin has no action upon sugar. When sugar is eaten there is a copious flow of saliva, but it contains no ptyalin. If soaked starches are eaten, no saliva is poured out upon these. Ptyalin is not poured out upon flesh or fat. These evidences of adaptation are but a few of the many that could be given. It seems probable that a wider range of adaptation is possible in gastric than in salivary secretion. These things are not without their significance to the person who is desirous of eating in a manner to assure most efficient digestion, although it is the custom of physiologists to gloss over or minimize them. We shall have occasion to refer to these matters in greater detail in subsequent chapters.

There are reasons for believing that man, like the lower animals, once instinctively avoided wrong combinations of foods, and there are remnants of the old instinctive practices still extant. But having kindled the torches of intellect upon the ruins of instinct, man is compelled to seek out his way in a bewildering maze of forces and circumstances by the fool's method of trial and error. At least this is so until he has gained sufficient knowledge and a grasp of proved principles to enable him to govern his conduct in the light of principles and knowledge. Instead, then, of ignoring the great mass of laboriously accumulated physiological knowledge relating to the digestion of our foodstuffs, or glossing over them as is the practice of the professional physiologists, it behooves us, as intelligent beings, to make full and proper use of such knowledge. If the physiology of digestion can lead us to eating practices that insure better digestion, hence better nutrition, only the foolish will disregard its immense value to us, both in health and in disease.

CHAPTER III

Right and Wrong Combinations

To make fully clear what combinations of foodstuffs override our enzymic limitations it will be necessary to consider, one by one, the possible combinations and briefly discuss these in their relations to the facts of digestion which we learned in the previous chapter. Such a study should prove both interesting and instructive to the intelligent reader.

ACID-STARCH COMBINATIONS

In the last chapter we learned that a weak acid will destroy the ptyalin of the saliva. With the destruction of the ptyalin starch digestion must come to a halt. The physiologist Stiles says: "If the mixed food is quite acid at the outset, it is hard to see how there can be any hydrolysis (enzymic digestion of starch) brought about by the saliva. Yet we constantly eat acid fruits before our breakfast cereal and notice no ill effects. Starch which escapes digestion at this stage is destined to be acted upon by the pancreatic juice, and the final result may be entirely satisfactory. Still it is reasonable to assume that the greater the work done by the saliva, the lighter will be the task remaining for the other secretions and the greater the probability of its complete accomplishment."

Howell says it appears that "this lipase is readily destroyed by an acidity of 0.2 per cent HC1, so that if it is of functional importance in gastric digestion its action, *like ptyalin, must be confined to the early period of digestion before the contents of the stomach have reached their normal acidity.*" (Italics mine.)

Oxalic acid diluted to 1 part in 10,000 completely arrests the action of ptyalin. There is sufficient acetic acid in one or two teaspoonfuls of vinegar to entirely suspend salivary digestion. The acids of tomatoes, berries, oranges, grapefruits, lemons, limes, pineapples, sour apples, sour grapes, and other sour fruits are sufficient to destroy the ptyalin of the saliva and suspend starch digestion. Without, apparently, understanding why, Dr. Percy Howe of Harvard, says: "Many people who cannot eat oranges at a meal derive great benefit from eating them fifteen to thirty minutes before the meal."

All physiologists agree that acids, even mild acids, destroy ptyalin. Unless and until it can be shown that saliva is capable of digesting starch without the presence of ptyalin, we shall have to continue to insist that acid-starch combinations are indigestible. The blatant assertion by men who never made a serious study of the subject of human nutrition, that any combination of foodstuffs that you like or desire is all right is based on ignorance or prejudice or is just an expression of bigotry.

Our rule, then, should be: *Eat acids and starches at separate meals.*

PROTEIN-STARCH COMBINATIONS

Chittednen showed that free hydrochloric acid to the extent of only 0.003 per cent is sufficient to suspend the starch-splitting (amylolytic) action of ptyalin, and a slight further increase in acidity not only stops the action, but also destroys the enzyme. In his *Textbook of Physiology* Howell says of *gastric lipase* that, "this lipase is readily destroyed by an acidity of 0.2 per cent HCl, so that if it is of functional importance in gastric digestion its action, like that of ptyalin, must be confined to the early period of digestion before the contents of the stomach have reached their normal acidity." We are not here concerned with the destruction of the *lipase* by the hydrochloric acid of the stomach, but with the destruction of ptyalin by the same acid.

The physiologist Stiles says: "the acid which is highly favorable to gastric digestion, for example, is quite prohibitive to salivary digestion." He says of pepsin, "the power to digest proteins is manifested only with an acid reaction, and is permanently lost when the mixture is made distinctly alkaline. The conditions which permit peptic digestion to take place are, therefore, precisely those which exclude the action of saliva." He declares of the salivary enzyme, ptyalin, "the enzyme is extremely sensitive to acid. Inasmuch as the gastric juice is decidedly acid it used to be claimed that salivary digestion could not proceed in the stomach." Gastric juice destroys ptyalin and thereby stops starch digestion. This being true, how are we ever to digest our starch foods?

The answer to this question is found in the power of the digestive system to adapt its secretions to the digestive requirements of particular foods, providing, of course that we respect the limitations of this adaptive mechanism. Dr. Richard C. Cabot of Harvard, who was neither advocating nor combatting any special method of food combining, wrote: "When we eat carbohydrates the stomach secretes an *appropriate* juice, a gastric juice of different composition from that which it secretes if it finds proteins coming down. This is a response to the particular demand that is made on the stomach. It is one of the numerous examples of choice or intelligent guidance carried on by parts of the body which are ordinarily thought of as unconscious and having no soul or choice of their own." Here is the secret: *The stomach secretes a different kind of juice when we eat a starch food from what it secretes when we eat a protein food.*

Pavlov has shown that each kind of food calls forth a particular activity of the digestive glands; that the power of the juice varies with the quality of the food; that special modifications of the activity of the glands are required by different foods; that the strongest juice is poured out when most needed.

When bread is eaten little hydrochloric acid is poured into the stomach. The juice secreted upon bread is almost neutral in reaction. When the starch of the bread is digested, much hydrochloric acid is then poured into the stomach to digest the protein of the bread. The two processes—the digestion of starch and the digestion of protein—do not go on simultaneously with great efficiency. On the contrary, the secretions are nicely and minutely adjusted, both as to character and to timing, to the varying needs of the complex food substance.

Herein lies the answer to those who object to food combining because "nature combines various food substances in the same food." There is a great difference between the digestion of a *food,* however complex its composition, and the digestion of a *mixture of different foods.* To a single article of food that is a starch-protein combination, the body can easily adjust its juices, both as to strength and timing, to the digestive requirements of the food. But when two foods are eaten with different, even opposite digestive needs, this precise adjustment of juices to requirements becomes impossible. If bread and flesh are eaten together, instead of an almost neutral gastric juice being poured into the stomach during the first two hours of digestion, a highly acid juice will be poured out immediately and starch digestion will come to an almost abrupt end.

It should never be lost sight of that physiologically, the first steps in the digestion of starches and proteins take place in opposite media—starch requiring an alkaline medium, protein requiring an acid medium in which to digest. On this point, V. H. Mottram, professor of physiology in the University of London, says in his *Physiology* that, when the food in the stomach comes in contact with the gastric juice, no salivary digestion is possible. He says: "Now gastric juice digests protein and saliva digests starch. Therefore it is obvious that for efficient digestion the meat (protein) part of a meal should come first and the starch part second—just indeed as by instinct is usually the case. Meat precedes pudding as being the most economical procedure."

Mottram explains this matter by saying: "The distal end of the stomach is that in which the churning movement that mixes the food with the gastric juice takes place. . . But the food in the quiescent end is still under the influence of the saliva, while the food in the motile end comes in contact with the acid gastric juice and no salivary action is possible." This simply means that if you eat your protein first and your starch last, that the protein will digest in the lower end of the stomach while the starch will digest in is upper end.

If we assume that there is any line of demarkation between the food in the stomach, as his proposition demands, it is still true that, people in general, neither instinctively nor otherwise, consume their proteins and starches in this manner. Perhaps in England it is customary to eat meat at the beginning of a meal and pudding at the end, just as we have a similar practice of taking a dessert at the end of a meal in this country, but it is likely to be the practice there as here, to eat starch and protein together. When the average man or woman eats flesh, or eggs, or cheese, he or she takes bread with the protein. Hot-dogs, ham sandwiches, hamburgers, toast and eggs, "ham on rye" and similar combinations of protein and starch represent the common practice of eating such foods. With such eating, the protein and starch are thoroughly mixed in both ends of the stomach.

Howell makes a somewhat similar statement. He says: "A question of practical importance is as to how far salivary digestion affects the starchy foods under usual circumstances. The chewing process in the mouth thoroughly mixes the food and saliva, or should do so, but the bolus is swallowed much too quickly to enable the enzyme to complete its action. In the stomach the gastric juice is sufficiently acid to destroy the ptyalin, and it was therefore supposed formerly that salivary digestion is promptly arrested on the entrance of food into the stomach, and is normally of but little value as a digestive process. Later knowledge regarding the conditions of the stomach shows, on the contrary, that some of the food in an ordinary meal may remain in the fundic end of the stomach for an hour or more untouched by the acid secretion. There is every reason to believe, therefore, that salivary digestion may be carried on in the stomach to an important extent."

It is obvious that salivary digestion may be carried on in the stomach to an important extent only in a small part of the food eaten, providing the eating is the usual haphazard mixtures of bread with meat, bread with eggs, bread with cheese, bread with other protein, or potatoes with proteins. When one eats a hamburger or a hot dog, one does not eat his flesh first and then follow with his bun. They are eaten together and thoroughly chewed and mixed together and swallowed together. The stomach has no mechanism for separating these thoroughly intermixed substances and partitioning them off in separate compartments in its cavity.

Mixing foods in this manner is not seen in nature—animals tending to eat but one food at a meal. The carnivore certainly does not mix starches with his proteins. Birds tend to consume insects at one period of the day and seeds at another time. This is certainly the best plan for man to follow, for, at best, the plan suggested by Mottram cannot give ideal results.

On the basis of the physiological facts which have been here presented, we offer our second rule for food combining. It is this: *Eat protein foods and carbohydrate foods at separate meals.*

By this is meant that cereals, bread, potatoes and other starch foods, should be eaten separately from flesh, eggs, cheese, nuts and other protein foods.

PROTEIN-PROTEIN COMBINATIONS

Two proteins of different character and different composition, and associated with other and different food factors call for different modifications of the digestive secretions and different timing of the secretions in order to digest them efficiently. For example, the strongest juice is poured out upon milk in the last hour of digestion, upon flesh in the first hour. Is there no significance in the timing of the secretions thus seen? In our eating practices we habitually ignore such facts and our physiologists have not attached any importance to such matters. Eggs receive the strongest secretion at a different time to that received by either flesh or milk. It is logical, therefore, to assume that eggs should not be taken with flesh or milk. It is not too late to recall the harm that was done to tubercular patients by feeding them the abominable combination of eggs and milk. It may be noted in passing that for centuries orthodox Jews have refrained from taking flesh and milk at the same meal.

The fact is that the digestive process is modified to meet the digestive requirements of each protein food and it is impossible for this to be modified in such a manner as to meet the requirements of two different proteins at the same meal. This may not mean that two different kinds of flesh may not be taken together or that two different kinds of nuts may not be taken at the same time; but it certainly means that such protein combinations as flesh and eggs, flesh and nuts, flesh and cheese, eggs and milk, eggs and nuts, cheese and nuts, milk and nuts, etc., should not be taken. One protein food at a meal will certainly assure greater efficiency in digestion.

Our rule, then, should be: *Eat but one concentrated protein food at a meal.*

An objection has been offered to this rule that is as follows: the various proteins vary so greatly in their amino-acid content and the body requires adequate quantities of certain of these so that, it is necessary to consume more than one protein in order to assure an adequate supply of amino-acids. But inasmuch as most people eat more than one meal a day and there is protein in almost everything we eat, this objection is invalid. One does not have to consume all of his protein at any one meal.

ACID-PROTEIN COMBINATIONS

The active work of splitting up (digesting) complex protein substances into simpler substances, which takes place in the stomach and which forms the first step in the digestion of proteins, is accomplished by the enzyme, *pepsin.* Pepsin acts only in an medium; its action is stopped by alkali. The gastric juice ranges all the way from nearly neutral to strongly acid, depending upon what kind of food is put into the stomach. When proteins are eaten the gastric juice is acid, for it must furnish a favorable medium for the action of *pepsin.*

Because pepsin is active only in an acid medium, the mistake has been made of assuming that the taking of acids with the meal will assist in the digestion of protein. Actually, on the contrary, these acids inhibit the outpouring of gastric juice and thus interfere with the digestion of proteins. Drug acids and fruit acids demoralize gastric digestion, either by destroying the *pepsin,* or by inhibiting its secretion. Gastric juice is not poured out in the presence of acid in the mouth and stomach. The renowned Russian physiologist, Pavlov, positively demonstrated the demoralizing influence of acids upon digestion—both fruit acids and the acid end-results of fermentation. Acid fruits by inhibiting the flow of gastric juice—an unhampered flow of which is imperatively demanded by protein digestion—seriously handicaps protein digestion and results in putrefaction.

The normal stomach secretes all the acid required by *pepsin* in digesting a reasonable quantity of protein. An abnormal stomach may secrete too much acid (hyperacidity) or an insufficient amount (hypoacidity). In either case, taking acids with proteins does not aid digestion. While *pepsin* is not active except in the presence of hydrochloric acid (I can find no evidence that other acids activate this enzyme), excessive gastric acidity prevents its action. Excess acid destroys the *pepsin.* Based on these simple facts of the physiology of digestion, our rule should be: *Eat proteins and acids at separate meals.*

When we consider the actual process of protein digestion in the stomach and the positive inhibiting effects of acids upon gastric secretion, we realize at once the fallacy of consuming pineapple juice or grapefruit juice or tomato juice with meat, as advocated by certain so-called dietitians, and the fallacy of beating up eggs in orange juice to make the so-called "pep-cocktail," advocated by other pseudo-dietitians.

Lemon juice, vinegar or other acid used on salads, or added to salad dressing, and eaten with a protein meal, serve as a severe check to hydrochloric secretion and thus interfere with protein digestion.

Although nuts or cheese with acid fruits do not constitute ideal combinations, we may make exceptions to the foregoing rule in the case of these two articles of food. Nuts and cheese containing, as they do considerable oil and fat (cream), are about the only exceptions to the rule that *when acids are taken with protein, putrefaction occurs.* These foods do not decompose as quickly as other protein foods when they are not immediately digested. Furthermore, acids do not delay the digestion of nuts and cheese; because these foods contain enough fat to inhibit gastric secretion for a longer time than do acids.

FAT-PROTEIN COMBINATIONS

Mcleod's *Physiology in Modern Medicine* says: "Fat has been shown to exert a distinct inhibiting influence on the secretion of gastric juice... the presence of oil in the stomach delays the secretion of juice poured out on a subsequent meal of otherwise readily digestible food." Here is an important physiological truth, the full significance of which has seldom been realized. Most men and women who write on food combining ignore the depressing effect fat has upon gastric secretion. The presence of fat in the food lessens the amount of appetite secretion that is poured into the stomach, lessens the amount of "chemical secretion" poured out, lessens the activity of the gastric glands, lowers the amount of pepsin and hydrochloric acid in the gastric juice and may lower gastric tone by as much as fifty per cent. This inhibiting effect may last two or more hours.

This means that when protein food is eaten, fat should not be taken at the same meal. In other words, such foods as cream, butter, oils of various kinds, gravies, fat meats, etc., should not be consumed at the same meal with nuts, cheese, eggs, flesh. It will be noted, in this connection, that those foods that normally contain fat within themselves, as nuts or cheese or milk, require longer time to digest than those protein foods that are lacking in fat.

Our fourth rule, then, is: *Eat fats and proteins at separate meals.*

It is well to know that an abundance of green vegetables, especially uncooked ones, counteract the inhibiting effect of fat, so that if one must have fat with one's protein, one may offset its inhibiting effect upon the digestion of protein by consuming much green substance with the meal.

SUGAR-PROTEIN COMBINATION

All sugars—commercial sugars, syrups, sweet fruits, honey, etc.—have an inhibiting effect upon the secretion of gastric juice and upon the motility of the stomach. This fact adds significance to the remark made to children by mothers that the eating of cookies before meals "spoils the appetite." Sugars taken with proteins hinder protein digestion.

Sugars undergo no digestion in the mouth and stomach. They are digested in the intestine. If taken alone they are not held in the stomach long, but are quickly sent into the intestine. When eaten with other foods, either proteins or starches, they are held up in the stomach for a prolonged period, awaiting the digestion of the other foods. While thus awaiting the completion of protein or starch digestion they undergo fermentation.

Based on these simple facts of digestion, our rule is: *Eat sugars and proteins at separate meals.*

SUGAR-STARCH COMBINATIONS

Starch digestion normally begins in the mouth and continues, under proper conditions, for some time in the stomach. Sugars do not undergo any digestion in either the mouth or stomach, but in the small intestine only. When consumed alone sugars are quickly sent out of the stomach into the intestine. When consumed with other foods, they are held up in the stomach for some time awaiting the digestion of the other foods. As they tend to ferment very quickly under the conditions of warmth and moisture existing in the stomach, this type of eating almost guarantees acid fermentation.

Jellies, jams, fruit butters, commercial sugar (white or brown, beet, cane or lactic), honey, molasses, syrups, etc., added to cakes, breads, pastries, cereals, potatoes, etc., *produce* fermentation. The regularity with which millions of our people eat cereals and sugar for breakfast and suffer with sour stomach, sour eructations, and other evidences of indigestion as a consequence, would be amusing were it not so tragic. Sweet fruits with starch also result in fermentation. Breads containing dates, raisins, figs, etc., so popular among the frequenters of the "health food" stores, are dietetic abominations. In many quarters it is thought that if honey is used instead of sugar this may be avoided, but such is not the case. Honey with hot cakes, syrup with hot cakes, etc., are almost sure to ferment.

There is every reason to believe that the presence of the sugar with the starch definitely interferes with the digestion of starch. When sugar is taken into the mouth there is a copious outpouring of saliva, but it contains no ptyalin for ptyalin does not act upon sugar. If the starch is disguised with sugar, honey, syrup, jellies, jams, etc., this will prevent the adaptation of the saliva to starch digestion. Little or no ptyalin will be secreted and starch digestion will not take place.

Major Reginald F. E. Austin, M.D., R.A.M.C., M.R.C.S., L.R.C.P., says: "foods that are wholesome by themselves or in certain combinations often disagree when eaten with others. For example, bread and butter taken together cause no unpleasantness, but if sugar or jam or marmalade is added trouble may follow. Because the sugar will be taken up first, and the conversion of the starch into sugar is then delayed. Mixtures of starch and sugar invite fermentation and its attendant evils."

Upon these facts we base the rule: *Eat starches and sugars at separate meals.*

EATING MELONS

Large numbers of people complain that melons do not agree with them. Some of these people, desiring to appear more up-to-date in their knowledge, explain that they are *allergic* to melons. I have fed melons in quantity to hundreds of such people and found that they have no trouble with them and that their supposed *allergy* was but a figment of the imagination. Melons are such wholesome foods and are so easy of digestion that even the most feeble digestions can handle them very nicely.

But trouble, frequently severe suffering, does often follow the eating of melons. Why? These foods undergo no digestion in the stomach. The little digestion they require takes place in the intestine. If taken properly, they are retained in the stomach but a few minutes and are then passed into the intestine. But if taken with other foods that require a lengthy stay in the stomach for salivary or gastric digestion, they are held up in the stomach. As they decompose very quickly when cut open and kept in a warm place, they are prone to give rise to much gas and discomfort when eaten with most other foods.

I take a patient who says that everytime he eats watermelon he has severe pain in his abdomen, that he fills up with gas, and that he suffers in other ways. He declares that melons have always "disagreed" with him, that he could never eat them. I feed this patient an abundance of melon and he has no gas, no pain, no discomfort. How do I achieve this? I feed the melon alone. He is given all the melon he desires at a meal—makes his meal on melon. He immediately discovers that melons do "agree" with him, that he is not *allergic* to melons.

From these facts we derive the rule: *Eat melons alone.*

This means that watermelons, honey dews, muskmelons, cantaloupes, casabas, Persian melons, banana melons, Crenshaw melons, pie melons, Christmas melons, and other melons should be eaten alone. They should not be eaten between meals, but at meal time. It is well to make the meal on melon.

I have tried feeding melons with fresh fruits and there seems to be no reason why they may not be fed together, if this is desired.

TAKE MILK ALONE

It is the rule in nature that the young of each species takes its milk alone. Indeed, in the early life of young mammals, they take no other food but milk. Then there comes a time when they eat milk and other foods, but they take them separately. Finally there comes a time when they are weaned, after which, they never take milk again. Milk is the food of the young. There is no need for it after the end of the normal suckling period. The dairy industry and the medical profession have taught us that we need a quart of milk a day so long as we live—we are never to be weaned but are to remain sucklings all our lives. This is a commercial program and expresses no human need.

Due to its protein and fat (cream) content, milk combines poorly with all foods. It will combine fairly well with acid fruits. The first thing that occurs when it enters the stomach is that it coagulates —forms curds. These curds tend to form around the particles of other food in the stomach thus insulating them against the gastric juice. This prevents their digestion until after the milk curd is digested.

Our rule with milk is: *Take milk alone or let it alone.*

In feeding milk to young children a fruit meal may be fed and then, half an hour afterward, milk may be given. The milk should not be given with the fruits, except in the case of acid fruits. The orthodox Jew follows a very excellent plan of eating when he refuses to consume milk with flesh. But its use with cereals or other starch is equally as objectionable.

DESSERTS

Desserts, eaten at the end of a meal, usually after the eater has eaten to repletion very commonly after he has eaten more than he requires of other foods, are such things as cakes, pies, puddings, ice cream, stewed fruits, etc.. which combine badly with almost every other part of the meal. They serve no useful purpose and are not advisable.

There should be but one rule with reference to them; it is this: *Desert the desserts.*

Dr. Tilden used to advise that if you must have a piece of pie, eat the pie and a large raw vegetable salad and nothing else and, then, *miss the next meal.* Dr. Harvey W. Wilev once remarked that the food value of pie is unquestioned: it only remains to be digested. Certainly, eaten with a regular meal, as is the custom, it is not well digested. The same may be said for the other desserts. Cold desserts, like ice cream, interpose another barrier to the digestive process-that of cold.

CHAPTER **IV**

Normal Digestion

In his *Textbook of Physiology* Howell says that "In the large intestine protein putrefaction is a constant and normal occurrence." He records that "Recognizing that fermentation by means of bacteria is a normal occurrence in the gastro-intestinal canal, the question has arisen whether this process is in any way necessary to normal digestion and nutrition." After considerable discussion of this question and reference to experiments that have been made he reaches no definite conclusion, but thinks "it seems wise to take the conservative view that while the presence of the bacteria confers no positive benefit, the organism has adapted itself under usual conditions to neutralize their injurious action."

He points out that the putrefactive bacteria break down the proteins into amino-acids, but that they do no stop here. They destroy the amino-acids and give us, as final products of their activities, such poisons as indol, skatol, phenol, phenylpropionie and phenylacetic acids, fatty acids, carbon dioxide, hydrogen, marsh gas, hydrogen sulphide, etc. He adds that "many of these products are given off in the feces, while others are absorbed in part and excreted subsequently in the urine." Finally, he says: "There is evidence that other more or less toxic substances belonging to the group of *amines* are produced by the further action of the bacteria on the aminoacids in the protein molecule."

It does not seem logical to assume that such a process of toxin formation is either normal or necessary in the process of digestion. It seems to me that Howell and the other physiologists have merely mistaken a common or almost universal occurrence, at least it is almost universal in civilized life, as a normal occurrence. They have not stopped to ask why fermentation and putrefaction occur in the digestive tract. What causes it to occur? That it is a source of poisoning they admit. Howell goes so far as to say: "It is well known that excessive bacterial action may lead to intestinal troubles, such as diarrhea, or possibly to more serious interference with nutrition owing to the formation of toxic products, such as the amines." He fails to define what he means by "excessive bacterial action."

I have repeatedly pointed out the folly of accepting mere conventions as normal. The mere fact that protein putrefaction is well-nigh universal in the colons of civilized man is, by itself, not sufficient to establish the phenomenon as a normal one. It is first necessary to ask and answer the question: *Why is protein putrefaction so common?* It may also be well to ask if it serves any useful purpose.

Are the putrefaction and fermentation that are so common due to overeating, to the eating of illegitimate proteins, to eating wrong combinations, to eating under physical and emotional conditions (fatigue, work, worry, fear, anxiety, pain, fever, inflammation, etc.) that retard or suspend digestion? Is it the result of impaired digestion from any cause? Must we always take it for granted that the present eating practices of civilized man are normal? Why must we accept as normal what we find in a race of sick and weakened beings?

Foul stools, loose stools, impacted stools, pebbly stools, much foul gas, colitis, hemorrhoids, bleeding with stools, the need for toilet paper, and all the other things of this nature that accompany present day living, are swept into the orbit of the normal by the assertion that putrefaction is a normal occurrence in the human colon. We have it asserted in different words that "whatever is, is right."

That there are animals that do not present protein putrefaction in their intestinal tracts, that there are men and women whose eating and living habits give odorless stools and no gas, that a change of habits produces a change of results—these facts are of no importance to physiologists who are devoted to the stultifying axiom that only conventions are to be received as data. Howell accepts as normal the generally prevailing septic condition of the human colon and completely ignores the causes that produce and maintain this condition of sepsis.

The blood stream should receive from the digestive tract water, amino-acids, fatty acids, glycerol, monosaccharides, minerals and vitamins. It should not receive alcohol, acetic acid, ptomaines, leucomaines, hydrogen sulphide, etc. Nutritive materials, not poisons, should be received from the digestive tract.

When starches and complex sugars are digested they are broken down into simple sugars called monosaccharides, which are usable substances—*nutriments.*

When starches and sugars undergo fermentation they are broken down into carbon dioxide, acetic acid, alcohol and water, which

substances, with the exception of water, are non-usable substances—
poisons. When proteins are digested, they are broken down into amino-acids, which are usable substances—nutrients. When proteins
putrefy, they are broken down into a variety of ptomaines and leucomaines, which are non-usable substances— *poisons.* So with all other
food factors—enzymic digestion of foods prepares them for use by the
body; bacterial decomposition of foods unfits them for use by the body.
The first process gives us nutrient elements as the finished product; the
second process gives us poisons as the end-result.

What avails it to consume the theoretically required number of calories daily, only to have the food ferment and putrefy in the digestive
tract? Food that thus spoils does not yield up its calories to the body.
What is gained by eating abundantly of adequate proteins only to have
these putrefy in the gastro-intestinal canal? Proteins thus rendered
unfit for entrance into the body do not yield up their amino-acids. What
benefit does one receive from eating vitamin-rich foods only to have
these decompose in the stomach and intestines? Foods thus rotted do not
supply the body with vitamins. What nutritive good comes from eating
mineral-laden foods only to have these rot in the alvine canal? Foods
that are thus rendered unfit for use provide the body with no minerals.
Carbohydrates that ferment in the digestive tract are converted into
alcohol and acetic acid, not into monosaccharides. Fats that become
rancid in the stomach and intestine provide the body with no fatty acids
and glycerol. To derive sustenance from the foods eaten, they must be
digested; they must not rot.

Discussing phenol, indol and skatol, Howell points out that phenol
(carbolic acid) after it is absorbed, is combined in part, with sulphuric
acid, forming an ethereal sulphate, or phenolsulphonic acid, and is
excreted in the urine in this form. "So also with cresol," he adds.
Indol and skatol, after being absorbed, are oxidized into indoxyl and
skatoxyl, after which they are combined with sulphuric acid, like phenol, and are excreted in the urine as indoxyl-sulphuric acid and ska-
toxyl-sulphuric acid. These poisons have long been found in the urine
and the amount of them occuring in the urine is taken as an index to
the extent of putrefaction that is going on in the intestine. That the
body may and does establish toleration for these poisons, as it does
for other poisons that are habitually introduced into it is certain, but
it seems the height of folly to assume that "the organism has adapted
itself under usual conditions to neutralize" these products of bacterial
activity. Certainly the discomfort that arises from the accumulation
of gas in the abdomen, the bad breath that grows out of gastro-intestinal fermentation and putrefaction, the foul and unpleasant odor

from the stools and from the expelled gasses are as undesirable as are the poisons.

That it is possible to have a clean sweet breath, freedom from gas pressure and odorless stools is common knowledge. It seems to me that instead of assuming that a common phenomenon is normal, perhaps even necessary, it were wise to consider the causes of this occurrence and determine whether or not it is normal. If it is possible to avoid the unpleasant results of fermentation and putrefaction, if it is possible to avoid the poisoning that results from these, if we can remove from the body the burden of oxydizing and eliminating these bacterial products, it seems to me to be eminendy desirable to do so. If it is admitted that "excessive bacterial activity" may produce diarrhea and even serious nutritional evils, what may we expect from long continued bacterial activity that is short of "excessive"? This, it seems to me, is a pertinent question.

Anything that reduces digestive power, anything that slows up the processes of digestion, anything that temporarily suspends the digestive process will favor bacterial activity. Such things as over eating (eating beyond enzymic capacity), eating when fatigued, eating just before beginning work, eating when chilled or over heated, eating when feverish, in pain, when there is severe inflammation, when not hungry, when worried, anxious, fearful, angry, etc.—eating under all of these and similar circumstances favors bacterial decomposition of the foods eaten. The use of condiments, vinegar, alcohol, and other substances that retard digestion favors bacterial activity. If we carefully analyze the eating practices of most civilized people, we may easily find a hundred and one reasons why gastro-intestinal fermentation and putrefaction are so nearly universal without assuming that these processes are normal, perhaps necessary. The causes of digestive inefficiency and failure are legion.

One of the most common causes of digestive inefficiency, one that is almost universally practiced in this country, is eating wrong combinations of foods. The almost universal practice of ignoring our enzymic limitations and eating haphazardly is responsible for a large part of the indigestion with which almost everybody suffers more or less constantly. The proof of this lies in the fact that feeding correct combinations ends the indigestion. This statement should not be misunderstood. Feeding correct combinations will only improve and not end indigestion, if the indigestion is due in part to other causes. If worry, for example, is a prominent factor in cause, worry will have to be discontinued before digestion can be normal. But it should be known that worry with wrong combinations will give worse indigestion than worry with correct combinations.

Rex Beach, who once mined gold in Alaska, wrote of gold miners: "We ate greatly of baking-powder bread, underdone beans and fat pork. No sooner were these victuals down than they went to war on us. The real call of the wild was not the howl of the timber wolf, the maniac laughter of the Artie loon, or the mating cry of the bull moose; it was the dyspeptic belch of the miner." Our physiologists, ignoring the mode of eating that is responsible for it, would declare this "belch of the miner," his abdominal distension and distress, the resulting gastro-intestinal decomposition, foul stools and passing of much foul gas, to be normal. If the miner did not have Bell-ans or Alkaseltzer with which to palliate his distress and encourage further indiscretions in eating, he could always run his finger down his throat and induce vomiting, if his distress became too great. Constipation, alternating with diarrhea, was common on such a diet.

Millions of dollars are spent yearly for drugs which afford a temporary respite from the discomfort and distress that result from decomposition of food in the stomach and intestine. Substances to neutralize acidity, to absorb gas, to relieve pain, even to relieve headache due to gastric irritation, are employed by train loads by the American people. Other substances, such as pepsin, are employed to aid in the digestion of food. Instead of regarding this as a normal condition, *Hygienists* regard it as an extremely abnormal condition. Ease and comfort, not pain and distress, are marks of health. Normal digestion is not accompanied with any signs or symptoms of disease.

Chapter V

How to Take Your Proteins

As all physiologists are agreed that the character of the digestive juice secreted corresponds with the character of the food to be digested and that each food calls for its own specific modification of the digestive juice, it follows as the night the day, that complex mixtures of foods greatly impair the efficiency of digestion. Simple meals will prove to be more easily digested, hence more healthful.

Conventional eating habits violate all of the rules of food combining that have been given in the preceding chapter and, since the majority of people manage to live for at least a few years and to "enjoy" their aches and pains and their frequent "spells of sickness," few of them are willing to give any intelligent consideration to their eating habits. They usually declare, when the subject of food combining comes up, that they eat all of the condemned combinations regularly and it does not hurt them. Life and death, health and disease are mere matters of accident to them. Unfortunately they are encouraged in this view by their medical advisers.

More than thirty years spent in feeding the well and the sick, the weak and the strong, the old and the young, have demonstrated that a change to correctly combined meals is followed by an immediate improvement in health as a consequence of lightening the load the digestive organs have to carry, thus assuring better digestion, improved nutrition and less poisoning. I know that such meals are followed by less fermentation and less putrefaction, less gas and discomfort. I do not believe that such experiences are worth much if they cannot be explained by correct principles, but I have explained them in preceding pages, so that they do assume great importance.

The rules of food combining herein given are soundly rooted in physiology, thoroughly tested by experience, and are worthy of more than a passing thought.

A great part of the yearly massacre of children's tonsils grows out of the constant fermentation in their digestive tracts consequent upon their regular eating a flesh-and-bread, cereals-and-sugar, cookies-and-fruit, etc. diet. Until parents learn how to feed their children with proper respect for enzymic limitations and cease feeding them the so-called "balanced meals" now in vogue, their children are going to continue to suffer, not only with colds and tonsillar troubles, but with gastritis (indigestion), diarrhea, constipation, feverishness, the various *children's diseases,* poliomyelitis, etc.

Commonly eaten combinations are bread and flesh—hot dogs, sandwiches, hamburgers, ham on rye, and the like—bread and eggs, bread and cheese, potatoes and flesh, potatoes and eggs, (eggs in a potato salad, for example), cereals with eggs (usually at breakfast), etc. Nor is it customary to eat the protein first and the carbohydrate afterwards. These foods are eaten together and thrown into the stomach in the most haphazard and indiscriminate manner. The customary way of eating breakfast is to have cereal first (usually with milk or cream and sugar), and then egg on toast. Viewing the common breakfast, which follows a common pattern eaten by most Americans, we should not be surprised that it is so regularly followed by indigestion, nor that the traffic in Bromo-Seltzer, Alkaseltzer, Bellans, Turns, baking soda, etc., is carried out on such a large scale.

Dishes of Italian origin that are growing very popular in this country are such mixtures as spaghetti and meat balls, spaghetti and cheese, spaghetti and ravioli. The spaghetti is commonly served with tomato sauce and white bread. A small chopped salad that accompanies, contains olive oil, vinegar and great quantities of salt. Other dressings are often served with the salad. White bread is usually served with this abominable mixture. In the smaller places oleomargarine is served. Beer or wine frequently is taken with such a meal.

The radio hawker tells the poor victims of such unphysiological habits of eating that when he suffers with "acid indigestion," he should resort to some one or other of the popular palliatives—nobody ever hints that such palliation guarantees the continuance of the evil habits and assures the later development of serious trouble. "Great oaks from little acorns grow," runs the old copybook maxim, but in this principle is not recognized by those who presume to know.

Inasmuch as, physiologically, the first step in the digestion of starch and the first step in the digestion of protein takes place in opposite media—starch requiring an alkaline medium, protein requiring an acid medium—these two types of foods certainly should not be eaten at the same meal. It is well known to physiologists that undigested starch absorbs pepsin. This being true it is inevitable that the eating of starches and proteins at the same meal will retard protein digestion. Tests have shown, it is claimed, that this retardation is not great—protein digestion being retarded but four to six minutes, which is insignificant. There is reason to believe that these findings are faulty. For, if the only result of such a combination is a four to six minutes retardation of the digestion of protein, so much undigested protein should not be found in the stools of those who eat such mixtures. I am convinced that the interference with protein digestion is greater than the tests indicate. Those who object to efforts to properly combine our foods tend to focus attention on the protein and, using the results of these tests as the basis of their objection to the rule against mixing proteins and carbohydrataes, they studiously avoid all reference to the suspension of starch digestion that results from such mixtures.

Previously we learned that it is unwise to consume more than one kind of protein at a meal. This is true, not merely because it complicates and retards the digestive process, but also, because it leads to over eating of protein. At present the trend is to overemphasize the need for protein foods and to encourage overeating of these foods. I would like to enter a warning against this folly at this place and point out that it is a return to the dietary fallacies of half a century ago. Diet fads, indeed, seem to run in circles.

So different in character are the specific secretions poured out upon each different food that Pavlov speaks of "milk juice," "bread juice" and "meat juice." Two proteins of different character and different composition require different types of digestive juices and these juices, of different strength and character are poured" into the stomach at different times during the digestive process. Khizhin, one of Pavlov's co-workers, showed that the secretion response of the digestive glands is not "limited to the powers of the juice but extends to the rate of its flow, and also its total quantity." The character of the food eaten determines not only the digestive power of the juice secreted upon it, but also its total acidity—acidity is greatest with flesh, least with bread. There is also a marvelous adjustment of the juice as to timing, the strongest juice being poured out in the first hour with flesh, in the third hour with bread, in the last hour of digestion with milk.

Due to the fact that each separate kind of food determines a definite hourly rate of secretion and occasions characteristic limitations in the various powers of the juices, foods requiring marked differences in the digestive secretions, as, for example, bread and flesh, certainly should not be consumed at the same meal. Pavlov showed that five times as much pepsin is poured out upon bread as upon milk containing an amount of protein equivalent to that contained in the bread, while the nitrogen of flesh requires more pepsin than milk. These different kinds of foods received quantities of enzyme corresponding to the differences in their digestibility. Comparing equivalent weights, flesh requires the most and milk the least amount of gastric juice, but comparing equivalents of nitrogen, bread needs the most and flesh the least juice.

All of these facts are very well known to physiologists, but they have never attempted to make any practical application of them. Indeed, when they condescend to discuss them at all in relation to the practical problems of life (of eating), they tend to gloss over them and to provide flimsy reasons why the haphazard eating practices that are almost everywhere in vogue should be continued. They are inclined to regard the more immediate evil results of such imprudent eating as normal, as was shown in the previous chapter.

Due to the inhibiting effects of acids, sugars and fats upon digestive secretion, it is unwise to eat such foods with proteins. Suppose we consider these combinations briefly in the order given.

The inhibiting effect of fat (butter, cream, oils, oleomargarine, etc.) upon gastric secretion, which retards protein digestion for two hours or more, renders it inadvisable to consume fats with proteins. The presence of fat in fat meats, in fried meats and fried eggs, in milk, nuts and similar foods is the probable reason that these foods require longer to digest than do lean roasts or coddled or poached eggs. Fat meats and fried meats are particularly likely to give the eater trouble. We should make it a rule, therefore, not to eat fats of any kind with our protein

The inhibiting effect of fat upon gastric secretion may be counteracted by consuming a plentiful supply of green vegetables, particularly uncooked. Uncooked cabbage is particularly effective in this respect. For this reason, it were better to consume green vegetables with cheese and nuts than to consume acid fruits with them, even though, this latter is not particularly objectionable.

Sugars, by inhibiting both gastric secretion and gastric motility (movement of the stomach) interfere with the digestion of proteins. At the same time these food substances, which require no digestion in the mouth and stomach, are held up pending the digestion of the proteins, hence they undergo fermentation. Proteins should not be eaten at the same meal with sugars of any kind or character. Dr. Norman's experiments showed that taking cream and sugar after a meal delays the digestion of the meal altogether for several hours.

Acids of all kinds inhibit the secretion of gastric juice. They thus interfere with the digestion of proteins. The exceptions are cheese, nuts and avocados. These foods, containing, as they do, cream and oil which inhibit the secretion of gastric juice as much and as long as do acids, do not have their digestion appreciably interfered with when acids are taken with them. The foods that combine best with protein foods of all kinds are the non-starchy and succulent vegetables. Spinach, chard, kale, beet greens, mustard greens, turnip greens, Chinese cabbage, broccoli, cabbage, asparagus, fresh green beans, okra, Brussell sprouts, all fresh tender squash, except Hubbard squash, onions, celery, lettuce, cucumbers, radishes, sorrel, water cress, parsley, endive, dandelion, collards, rape, escarole, cardoon, broccoli-de-rappe, bamboo sprouts and similar non-starchy foods.

The following vegetables form poor foods to combine with proteins: beets, turnips, pumpkins, carrots, salsify (vegetable oyster or oyster plant), cauliflower, kohlrabi, rutabagas, beans, peas, Jerusalem artichokes, potatoes, including the sweet potato. Being somewhat starchy, they make better additions to the starch meal. Beans and peas, being protein-starch combinations in themselves, are better eaten as a starch or as a protein, combined with green vegetables, without other protein or starch with the meal. Potatoes are sufficiently starchy to form the starch part of the starch meal.

The following menus constitute properly combined protein meals. It is suggested that the protein meal be eaten in the evening. Acids and oils and oily dressings should not be taken with the protein meals. These meals may be eaten in amounts required by the individual.

Vegetable Salad	Vegetable Salad	Vegetable Salad
Green Squash	Collards	Spinach
Spinach	Yellow Squash	Green Squash
Nuts	Avocado	Cottage Cheese
Vegetable Salad	Vegetable Salad	Vegetable Salad
Chard	Mustard Greens	Beet Greens
Asparagus	String Beans	Green Peas
Nuts	Avocado	Cottage Cheese
Vegetable Salad	Vegetable Salad	Vegetable Salad
Broccoli	Yellow Squash	Spinach
Fresh Corn	Cabbage	Cabbage
Nuts	Sunflower Seed	Unprocessed Cheese
Vegetable Salad	Vegetable Salad	Vegetable Salad
Okra	Spinach	Baked Eggplant
Spinach	Broccoli	Chard
Nuts	Sunflower Seed	Eggs

Vegetable Salad
Chard
Yellow Squash
Nuts

Vegetable Salad
Chard
Okra
Cottage Cheese

Vegetable Salad
Spinach
Yellow Squash
Eggs

Vegetable Salad
Beet Greens
String Beans
Nuts

Vegetable Salad
Okra
Yellow Squash
Cottage Cheese

Vegetable Salad
Turnip Greens
String Beans
Eggs

Vegetable Salad
Chard
Yellow Squash
Lamb Chops

Vegetable Salad
Chard
Yellow Squash
Avocado

Vegetable Salad
Okra
Red Cabbage
Avocado

Vegetable Salad
Green Squash
Kale
Unprocessed Cheese

Vegetable Salad
White Cabbage
Spinach
Nuts

Vegetable Salad
Asparagus
Cone Artichokes
Avocado

Vegetable Salad
Beet Greens
Okra
Sunflower Seed

Vegetable Salad
Broccoli
Green Beans
Nuts

Vegetable Salad
Yellow Squash
Chard
Avocado

Vegetable Salad
Kale
String Beans
Sunflower Seed

Vegetable Salad
Steamed Onions
Swiss Chard
Unprocessed Cheese

Vegetable Salad
Baked Eggplant
Kale
Avocado

Vegetable Salad
Baked Eggplant
Chard
Soy Sprouts

Vegetable Salad
Green Squash
Turnip Greens
Roast Beef

Vegetable Salad
Yellow Squash
Mustard Greens
Pecans

Vegetable Salad
Asparagus
Green Beans
Walnuts

Vegetable Salad
Red Cabbage
Spinach
Cottage Cheese

Vegetable Salad
String Beans
Okra
Broiled Lamb

Vegetable Salad
Okra
Beet Greens
Sunflower Seed

Vegetable Salad
Asparagus
Broccoli
Eggs

Vegetable Salad
Brussel Sprouts
Kale
Nuts

Chapter VI

How to Take Your Starch

One author says: "Don't serve more than two foods rich in sugar or starch at the same meal. When you serve bread and potatoes, your starch-license has run out. A meal that includes peas, bread, potatoes, sugar, cake and after dinner mints should also include a Vitamin B Complex capsule, some bicarbonate of soda (other than that used on the vegetables), and the address of the nearest specialist in arthritis and other degenerative diseases."

For more than fifty years it has been the rule in Hygienic circles to take but one starch at a meal and to consume no sweet foods with the starch meal. Sugars, syrups, honey's cakes, pies, mints, etc., have been tabu with starches. We do not say to those who come to us for advice: If you eat these with your starches, take a dose of baking soda with them. We tell them to avoid the fermentation that is almost inevitable. In *Hygienic* circles it is considered the height of folly to take a poison and then take an antidote with it. We think it best not to take the poison.

Sugar with starch means fermentation. It means a sour stomach. It means discomfort. Those who are addicted to the honey-eating practice and who are laboring under the popular fallacy that honey is a "natural sweet" and may be eaten indiscriminately, should know that this rule not to take sweets with starches applies to honey as well. Honey or syrup, it makes no difference which, with your hot cakes, honey or sugar, it matters not which, with your cereals, honey or sugar to sweeten your cakes—these combinations spell fermentation.

White sugar, brown sugar, "raw" sugar, imitation brown sugar (that is, white sugar that has been colored), black strap molasses, or other syrup, with starches means fermentation. Soda will neutralize the resulting acids, it will not stop the fermentation.

For more than fifty years it has been the practice in *Hygienic* circles to take a large raw vegetable salad (leaving out tomatoes or other acid foods) with the starch meal. The salad has been a very large one, measured by ordinary standards, and made up of fresh uncooked vegetables. This salad carries an abundance of vitamins and minerals. The vitamins in these vegetables are the genuine articles and no chemist's imitations of the real thing. No just-as-good substitutes for vitamins have ever satisfied the *Hygienists*. We take the real article or nothing. Capsule-eating is a commercial program and belongs to the drug fetish.

Vitamins complement each other. We need, not just the vitamin B complex, but all vitamins. A large raw vegetable salad supplies several known vitamins and those that may exist but have not yet been detected. Vitamins not only cooperate with each other in the nutritive process, but they also cooperate with the minerals in the body. These are supplied by the vegetable salad. To take vitamin preparations that are combined with calcium or iron or other minerals will not answer the purpose. These minerals are in non-usable forms. There is no better source of food substances than the plant kingdom—the laboratory and the chemist have not yet been able to concoct acceptable foods.

Hygienists advise but one starch at a meal, not because there is any conflict in the digestion of these foods, but because taking two or more starches at a meal is practically certain to lead to overeating of this substance. We find it best, and this is doubly true in feeding the sick, to limit the starch intake to one starch at a meal. People with unusual powers of self-control may be permitted two starches, but these individuals are so rare, the rule should be: *one starch at a meal.*

The same author says: "Whether you eat hamburgers at the Greasy Spoon—or filet mignon at the Plaza—you're eating protein. Whether it's griddle cakes at the diner—or crepe suzette at the Astorbilt—you're eating carbohydrates. And whether its oleomargarine from a relief agency, or butter balls at the Cafe de Lux—you're eating fat. These are the big three; the fourth part of food is roughage. All food will predominate in one of these substances or another. Some highly refined foods—like sugar—will contain only one of these, but—generally speaking, most foods contain all three—which is what makes the Hay Diet somewhat elusive."

It is not true that the fourth part of food is roughage, for roughage is not food, and it is not true that all foods predominate in one or the other of these four "parts of foods." Young, tender, growing plants have very little roughage, their cellulose being practically all digestible. They are valuable largely for their minerals and vitamins. His "big four" does not take into account the minerals that are in foods, and which are very abundant in many foods, while relatively scarce in others.

One may easily get the idea, from reading the foregoing quotation, that one protein is as good as another, that one fat is as good as another, that any combination of food, such as hamburgers or filet mignon, is as good as any other, and that foods may be prepared in any manner desired. Its author is not actually guilty of holding any such views, but this statement of his could easily lead his readers to believe that just any old diet is good enough.

The remark that I wish to discuss is that, generally speaking, most foods contain carbohydrates, fats, proteins and roughage and that, this makes the prohibition of protein-starch combinations "somewhat elusive." I want to differentiate between natural food combinations and the haphazard combinations commonly eaten. The human digestive tract is adapted to the digestion of natural combinations, but it is certainly not adapted to the digestion of the haphazard and indiscriminate combinations that are eaten in civilized life today. Natural combinations offer but little difficulty to the digestive system; but, it is one thing to eat one food, however complex its nature; it is quite another thing to eat two foods of "opposite character." The digestive juices may be readily adapted to one food, such as cereals, that is a protein-starch combination; they cannot be well adapted to two foods, such as bread and cheese. Tilden frequently said that nature never produced a sandwich.

It should be axiomatic that our digestive system is adapted to the digestion of natural combinations and can handle the unnatural ones only with difficulty. Modern civilized eating habits are so far removed from anything seen anywhere in nature or among so-called primitive peoples that it is impossible to think of them as being normal eating habits.

The prohibition is "somewhat elusive" to him simply because he has not given enough attention to the process of digestion. It is true that Nature puts up such combinations. It is true that these natural combinations offer but little difficulty to digestion. But, and here is the fact of digestion that all orthodox dietitians miss, the body is capable of so adapting its digestive secretions, both as to strength of acid, concentration of enzymes and timing of secretions, to the digestive requirements of a particular food, while such precise adaptation of juices to foods is not possible when two different foods are eaten. Cannon demonstrated that if starch is well mixed with saliva, it will continue to digest in the stomach for as much as two hours. This certainly cannot be true if proteins are eaten with the starch, for, in this case, the glands of the stomach will deluge the food with an acid gastric juice, thus rapidly ending gastric salivary digestion.

He says that the purpose of saliva is to begin the process of digestion of starches. "That is why," he adds, "you should chew bread, cereals, and other starchy foods very thoroughly; that is why you must not drink water through a mouthful of food. Though water at meal time is not condemned—it is needed to help the body in the chemistry of digestion—it must not be permitted to weaken the action of saliva on starches in the mouth."

The digestion of starches begins in the mouth, or should, but they remain in the mouth for such a short time that very little digestion takes place. Salivary digestion of starches can and will continue in the stomach for a long period if they are eaten under proper conditions. Eating acids and proteins with them will inhibit or completely suspend their digestion. Drinking water with the meal will weaken the action of saliva upon starches in the stomach as much as it will in the mouth, and it is not true that you need to drink at meal time to have water to aid in the digestion of your food. It will be best to drink your water ten to fifteen minutes before meals. If taken with meals it dilutes the digestive juices and then passes out of the stomach in short order carrying the digestive juices and their enzymes along with it. The following menus constitute properly combined starch meals. It is suggested that the starch meal be eaten at noon time. Starches should be eaten dry and should be thoroughly chewed and insalivated before swallowing. Acids should not be eaten on the salad with the starch meal. We suggest a larger salad in the evening with the protein and a smaller one at noon with the starch. These menus may be eaten in amounts required by the individual.

Vegetable Salad	Vegetable Salad	Vegetable Salad
Turnip Greens	Spinach	Beet Greens
Yellow Squash	Red Cabbage	Okra
Chestnuts	Baked Caladium Roots	Brown Rice
Vegetable Salad	Vegetable Salad	Vegetable Salad
Spinach	String Beans	Turnip Greens
String Beans	Steamed Egg Plant	Asparagus
Coconut	Steamed Caladium Roots	Brown Rice
Vegetable Salad	Vegetable Salad	Vegetable Salad
String Beans	Turnip Greens	Collards
Mashed Rutabagga	Okra	Fresh Corn
Irish Potatoes	Jerusalem Artichoke	Brown Rice

Vegetable Salad
Spinach
Beets
Irish Potatoes

Vegetable Salad
Kale
Okra
Jerusalem Artichoke

Vegetable Salad
Beet Greens
Cauliflower
Baked Hubbard
    Squash

Vegetable Salad
Chard
Carrots
Potatoes

Vegetable Salad
Chard
Yellow Squash
Jerusalem Artichoke

Vegetable Salad
Kale
String Beans
Baked Hubbard
    Squash

Vegetable Salad
String Beans
Turnips
Sweet Potatoes

Vegetable Salad
Spinach
Turnips
Jerusalem Artichoke

Vegetable Salad
Green Squash
Okra
Baked Hubbard
    Squash

Vegetable Salad
Asparagus
White Squash
Yams

Vegetable Salad
Okra
String Beans
Jerusalem Artichoke

Vegetable Salad
Turnip Greens
Broccoli
Peanuts

Vegetable Salad
Beet Greens
Cauliflower
Sweet Potatoes

Vegetable Salad
Asparagus
Okra
Peanuts

Vegetable Salad
Swiss Chard
Peas
Hubbard Squash

Vegetable Salad
Chard
String Beans
Peanuts

Vegetable Salad
Okra
Beet Greens
Whole Grain Bread

Vegetable Salad
String Beans
Broccoli
Hubbard Squash

Vegetable Salad
Spinach
Green String Beans
Brown Rice

Vegetable Salad
Yellow Wax Beans
Kale
Irish Potatoes

Vegetable Salad
Spinach
Cabbage
Baked Hubbard
    Squash

Vegetable Salad
Chard
Okra
Brown Rice

Vegetable Salad
String Beans
Yellow Squash
Irish Potatoes

Vegetable Salad
Beet Greens
Yellow Squash
Irish Potatoes

Vegetable Salad
Chard
Asparagus
Baked Beans

Vegetable Salad
Okra
Brussell Sprouts
Irish Potatoes

Vegetable Salad
Kale
Okra
Brown Rice

Vegetable Salad
Swiss Chard
Yellow Squash
Baked Caladium
    Roots

Vegetable Salad
String Beans
Cabbage
Sweet Potatoes

Vegetable Salad
Chard
Broccoli
Yams

Vegetable Salad
Spinach
String Beans
Peanuts

Vegetable Salad
Okra
Beet Greens
Steamed Caladium
    Roots

Vegetable Salad
Spinach
Cabbage
Chestnuts

Vegetable Salad
Okra
Cauliflower
Carrots

Vegetable Salad
Yellow Squash
Chard
Potatoes

CHAPTER VII

Eating Fruits

William Henry Porter, M.D. says in his book, *Eating to Live Long,* that eating fruits "is one of the most pernicious and reprehensible of dietetic follies." But he admits that fruits eaten without other foods are all right. I doubt not that if he were approached on the subject of food combining, he would declare it to be a pernicious fad. Dr. Percy Howe of Harvard noted that people who could not eat oranges with meals were able to eat them alone without trouble. Dr. Dewey, of fasting fame, was strongly opposed to the eating of fruits, declaring that they demoralize digestion. None of these men knew anything of food combining. They merely noted that eating fruits with other foods results in a large amount of trouble, hence, they condemned, not the other foods, but the fruits. Actually, there is no more reason to condemn the fruit than there is to condemn the other food with which the fruit is taken.

Man, the archtype of the *cheirotheria*, should develop those frugivorous habits which are common to his anatomical structure, and from which he has largely departed in the course of time, due, no doubt in large measure to his wanderings since he left his edenic home in the warmer regions. His sense of taste, being the expression of organic demand, must, of course, share in his health or his disease, and the taste which now demands flesh, will give place to a more exquisite appreciation of savors in the great varieties of fruits, vegetables and nuts in their many, varied and artistic combinations, which appeal as much to the eye and nose as to the tongue.

Fruits are among the finest and best of foods. Nothing affords us more good eating pleasure than a rich, mellow apple, a luscious, well-ripened banana, a carefully selected buttery, creamy, smooth avocado, or the wholesome, heart-warming goodness of a sweet grape. Real gustatory happiness is derived from the peach brought to the point of ripe perfection. Fruits, indeed, are a taste-enchanting, treasure trove of delightful eating enjoyment. With their luxury blends of rare flavors, delightful aromas, eye-pleasing colors, fruits are always an invitation to pleasure in eating.

Fruits are more than just a delight to the eye, the nose and the mouth—they are master mixtures of pure, rich, real food elements. Few of them are rich in protein—the avocado and olive being the chief exceptions—but are packed full of mouth-watering sugars; are all-star flavor blends of acids, are full of minerals and vitamins. Together with nuts (which, botanically, are also classed as fruits) and green vegetables, fruits constitute an adequate diet—indeed, these foods constitute the ideal diet of the normally frugivorous animal: man.

Fruit eating affords us much deep-down pleasure. Mother nature has flavored them just right to afford us the greatest enjoyment in eating. They are just right for our taste contentment. There is every reason why we should eat these foods with which mother nature so compellingly entices us to eating enjoyment and which she has filled with so much pure, rich, wholesome nourishment.

Nothing can afford us more gustatory happiness and real deep down taste contentment than a meal of luscious fruits. Such a meal is always an invitation to pleasure. A fruit meal will not cause the troubles that flow from eating fruits with other foods. Such a meal will not demoralize digestion. It will do most for you. It is both refreshing and nourishing. The exquisite delight of eating such a naturally good meal, the wonderful feeling of comfort that follows, the real, genuine satisfaction it affords, far surpass that of eating other foods.

And this is the ideal manner in which to eat your fruits. Eat them at a fruit meal. The acids of fruits do not combine well with either starches or proteins; their sugars do not combine with either proteins or starches, the oils of the avocado and olive do not combine well with protein. Why risk digestive trouble by eating such foods with flesh, eggs, bread, etc.

Fruits undergo little or no digestion in the mouth and stomach and are, as a rule quickly sent into the intestine, where they undergo the little digestion they require. To eat them with other foods that do require considerable time in the stomach is to have them held up there pending the completion of the digestion of the other foods. Bacterial decomposition follows. We have previously considered this fact with reference to melons which are also fruits.

Fruits should not be eaten between meals. To eat them between meals is to put them into the stomach while the stomach is still busily engaged in digesting the previous meal. Trouble is sure to follow. Our rule, one from which we will do well not to vary, is to *eat fruit at a fruit meal.*

The habit of drinking quantities of fruit juices—lemon juice, orange juice, grapefruit juice, grape juice, tomato juice, papaya juice —between meals is responsible for a large amount of indigestion in those who think they are eating healthfully. This practice, revived during the last few years, was quite the vogue in *Hygienic* circles sixty to eighty years ago, and the digestive and other evils that flowed from it caused many to abandon the reform diet and return to their flesh pots. Let me recount Dr. Robert Walter's experience with the juice drinking fad, as he records it in his *Exact Science of Health.*

He says that in consequence of the treatments he had undergone in his efforts to recover health (first medical and then hydropathic), he had a "ravenous appetite for food" and as a consequence of the irritation of his stomach he had developed into a "gourmand which no amount of food could satisfy." He adds: "My sufferings from thirst were always great, but I did not like water, and having been taught the superior qualities of fruits, I could never get enough of the cooling juices, which fermented in my stomach, creating and perpetuating the very fever they temporarily relieved, all of which ***kept me in a fever of nervous hunger which no suffering in other respects ever equalled."

This experience caused the doctor to renounce vegetarianism and return to meat eating. Eating at all hours of the day (for drinking juices is eating), he developed a neurosis which he mistook for hunger. Trying to satisfy a neurosis by eating is like trying to put out a fire with gasoline. Those who mistake gastric irritation for hunger and who continue to "appease" their "hunger" with the use of the cause of the irritation must grow from bad to worse. Turning from vegetarianism saved Dr. Walter, not because vegetarianism is wrong, but because he began to eat but one meal a day and ceased to imbibe fruit juices between meals.

No diet is so good but that it will be spoiled by the juice drinking practice and no diet is so bad but that this practice will make it worse. And this is true, not because the juices are bad, for they are excellent, but because their use in such manner disorganizes digestion.

Many mistakes that are now being made by so-called dietitians could be avoided if they were acquainted with the history of diet reform. All of their "discoveries" were made and tried long ago, and some of those that are just now enjoying a heyday of popularity, were found evil and abandoned.

Although green vegetables form the ideal combination with nuts, acid fruits form a fair combination with these foods and may be taken with them. This, of course, has reference to protein nuts and not to the starchy ones — coconuts, chestnuts, acorns, etc. Sweet fruits and nuts form a particularly objectionable combination, despite the delightful flavor of the mixture.

Avocados, containing more protein than milk, should not be combined with other proteins. Rich in fat, they also inhibit the digestion of other proteins. There can be no objection to combining them with acid fruits. They are best not eaten with sweet fruits. Nor should they be combined with nuts. In many quarters it is contended that the papaya assists in the digestion of proteins and we are strongly urged to eat it with proteins for this reason. Such a combination is not wise and, if it is true, as contended, that there is an enzyme in the papaya that will digest protein, it is an added reason not to combine it with protein. The employment of "aids to digestion" invariably weakens the patient's power of digestion. If his digestion is impaired, the sensible procedure is to remove the cause or causes of digestive impairment and then provide the digestive system with sufficient rest for repair and recuperation.

In feeding fruit meals to the sick I have found it best to feed sweet fruits and the strongly acid fruits at separate meals. Thus, I do not feed dates or figs or bananas with oranges or grapefruit, or pineapples. Sugar, honey or other sweets with grapefruit is particularly objectionable. If your grapefruit is bitter or excessively sour, get the naturally superior grapefruit from the lower Rio Grande Valley.

The following menus constitute properly combined fruits and it is suggested that the fruit meal be eaten for breakfast. Do not add sugar to the fruits. Any fruit in season may be used. These meals may be eaten in amounts required by the individual.

Oranges	Fresh Figs	Mangoes
Grapefruit	Peaches	Cherries
	Apricots	Apricots
Oranges	Cherries	Cherries
Pineapple	Apricots	Peaches
	Plums	Nectarines
Grapefruit	Bananas	Berries with Cream
Apples	Pears	(No sugar)
	Grapes	
Mangoes	Papaya	Bananas
Cherries	Persimmons	Persimmons
Apricots		Dates

Apples	Dates	Bananas
Grapes	Apples	Pear
Figs	Pears	Figs
		Glass of Sour Milk

As a variation, a very tasty meal may be made of a fruit salad and a protein as follows:

A large fruit salad composed of:

Grapefruit, orange, apple, pineapple, lettuce, celery.

Four ounces of cottage cheese or four ounces of nuts, or a greater amount of avocado.

In the Spring a tasty salad may be made of the fruits in season: peach, plum, apricot, cherry, nectarine, lettuce, celery.

Sweet fruits—bananas, raisins, dates, figs, prunes, etc.—should not be put into the salad when it is intended to have a protein with it.

CHAPTER VIII

Eating Schedule for a Week

All the menus given in this book are intended merely as guides to the reader to assist him in understanding the principles of food combining and to enable him to work out his own menus. It is my thought that it is more important to know how to make up one's own menus than to have a book of menus giving three meals a day for every day in the year. The person who understands food combining and who is able to arrange his own menus is never at a loss, wherever he is, in preparing his meals. He can devise a meal from the foods at hand.

The same foods are not always available in all parts of the country. A food that is available in one section of the country at one time of the year may be available in another part of the country at a different time of the year. Food availability varies with season, climate, altitude, soil and market facilities. The man who knows how to combine his meals may make use of the foods that are at hand and work out a meal. The man who depends on a cut and dried book of menus and does not know how to combine his foods may find that the particular foods listed in the menu for today are not available—he is left out on a limb. What he usually does is take the easy way and eat indiscriminately. If you are at the home of a friend or relative, your book of menus can be of no service to you; but if you know how to combine your foods, you may usually pick out compatible combinations from the foods spread before you and eat a well-combined meal.

Learn the principles of food combining so that you may properly apply them in any and all circumstances in which you may find yourself. A child may be able to follow a chart; an intelligent adult should learn principles and learn to apply these. Once you have done this and have practiced properly combining your foods for a time, the practice becomes automatic and you do not have to spend a lot of time on it.

Above all things, do not become a crank on the matter. Eat your meal and forget it. Let your friends eat their foods and don't give them a lecture on dietetics at the dining table

The following two weekly schedules are designed to demonstrate the proper ways to combine foods at different seasons of the year. The first week's schedule covers foods available in Spring and Summer. The second week's schedule covers foods available in Fall and Winter. Use these merely as guides and learn to prepare your own menus.

SPRING AND SUMMER MENUS

SUNDAY

BREAKFAST	LUNCH	DINNER
Watermelon	Vegetable Salad	Vegetable Salad
	Chard	String Beans
	Yellow Squash	Okra
	Potatoes	Nuts

MONDAY

BREAKFAST	LUNCH	DINNER
Peaches	Vegetable Salad	Vegetable Salad
Cherries	Beet Greens	Spinach
Apricots	Carrots	Cabbage
	Baked Beans	Cottage Cheese

TUESDAY

BREAKFAST	LUNCH	DINNER
Cantaloupes	Vegetable Salad	Vegetable Salad
	Okra	Broccoli
	Green Squash	Fresh Corn
	Jerusalem Artichokes	Avocado

WEDNESDAY

BREAKFAST	LUNCH	DINNER
Berries with Cream (No sugar)	Vegetable Salad	Vegetable Salad
	Cauliflower	Green Squash
	Okra	Turnip Greens
	Brown Rice	Lamb Chops

THURSDAY

BREAKFAST	LUNCH	DINNER
Nectarines	Vegetable Salad	Vegetable Salad
Apricots	Green Cabbage	Beet Greens
Plums	Carrots	String Beans
	Sweet Potatoes	Nuts

FRIDAY

BREAKFAST	LUNCH	DINNER
Watermelon	Vegetable Salad	Vegetable Salad
	Baked Eggplant	Yellow Squash
	Chard	Spinach
	Whole Wheat Bread	Eggs

SATURDAY

BREAKFAST	LUNCH	DINNER
Bananas	Vegetable Salad	Vegetable Salad
Cherries	Green Beans	Kale
Glass of Sour Milk	Okra	Broccoli
	Irish Potatoes	Soy Sprouts

FALL AND WINTER MENUS

SUNDAY

BREAKFAST	LUNCH	DINNER
Grapes	Vegetable Salad	Vegetable Salad
Bananas	Chinese Cabbage	Spinach
Dates	Asparagus	Yellow Squash
	Baked Caladium	Baked Beans
	Roots	

MONDAY

BREAKFAST	LUNCH	DINNER
Persimmons	Vegetable Salad	Vegetable Salad
Pear	Kale	Brussel Sprouts
Grapes	Cauliflower	String Beans
	Yams	Pecans

TUESDAY

BREAKFAST	LUNCH	DINNER
Apples	Vegetable Salad	Vegetable Salad
Grapes	Turnip Greens	Kale
Dried Figs	Okra	Yellow Squash
	Brown Rice	Avocado

WEDNESDAY

BREAKFAST	LUNCH	DINNER
Pears	Vegetable Salad	Vegetable Salad
Persimmons	Broccoli	Okra
Banana	String Beans	Spinach
Glass of Sour Milk	Irish Potato	Pignolias

THURSDAY

BREAKFAST	LUNCH	DINNER
Papaya	Vegetable Salad	Vegetable Salad
Orange	Green Squash	Red Cabbage
	Parsnips	String Beans
	Whole Grain Bread	Sunflower Seed

FRIDAY

BREAKFAST	LUNCH	DINNER
Persimmons	Vegetable Salad	Vegetable Salad
Grapes	Carrots	Chard
Dates	Spinach	Yellow Squash
	Steamed Caladium Roots	Unprocessed Cheese

SATURDAY

BREAKFAST	LUNCH	DINNER
Grapefruit	Vegetable Salad	Vegetable Salad
	Fresh Peas	Spinach
	Kale	Steamed Onions
	Coconut	Lamb Chops

SUNDAY

BREAKFAST	LUNCH	DINNER
Honey Dew Melon	Vegetable Salad	Vegetable Salad
	String Beans	Baked Eggplant
	Vegetable Soup	Kale
	Yams	Eggs

CHAPTER IX

Remedying Indigestion

It is impossible to overestimate the importance of good digestion. Upon the efficiency of the digestive process depends the preparation of the raw materials of nutrition; hence, upon good digestion depends, to a very large extent, the well-being of the body. There can be no such thing as good nutrition without good digestion. The best of diets fails to yield up its greatest good when the digestive process fails in the work of preparing it for use by the body.

Poor digestion cannot be depended upon to supply the materials with which to build and maintain good blood; hence the tissues will be inadequately nourished, the general health must fail and the constitution deteriorate. It is of great importance to remember that the normal process of blood making depends upon the first step in the preparation of blood-making materials in the digestive tract. Good digestion, therefore, means more normal tissue change throughout the body. Improved digestion results in general improvement in all of the functions of life. Many and great are the benefits to flow from improved digestion.

Indigestion is the forerunner, not the cause, of many of man's more serious ills. But every impairment of function becomes a secondary source of cause, and the poisoning and starvation that result from indigestion are added causes of suffering.

These are superadded to the primary causes of man's suffering. When indigestion is prevented health is preserved; when it is remedied health is restored.

A whole train of discomforts or symptoms accompany the progressive impairment of the function of digestion, such as gas, sour eructations, a sense of discomfort running into pain in the abdomen, sleepless and unrefreshing nights, furred tongue in the morning, absence of desire for food, constipation, foul stools, nervousness, etc. This is by no means an exhaustive catalogue of the symptoms that accompany indigestion.

If we reflect for a minute upon the enormous quantities of baking soda (bicarbonate of soda), milk of magnesia, Alka-seltzer, Bromo-seltzer, Turns, Bell-Anns, charcoal, and other drugs that are daily consumed by the American people to relieve them of distress arising out of acid fermentation and gas in the digestive tract, all of this growing out of indigestion, we may readily reach the conclusion that, as a people, we are suffering from indigestion. Distress after meals is exceedingly common and nobody seems to know how to do more than give the sufferers a few minutes to a few hours of respite from their distress. It is a sad commentary upon the much touted "science" of medicine that it can do nothing lasting or constructive in a simple functional condition of this nature.

Besides the drugs employed to temporarily allay distress, there are many "aids to digestion" in use. Pepsin is, perhaps, the best known of these. For a time, chewing gum was declared to aid the digestion of food. These "aids to digestion" are all frauds. They do not aid digestion at all. They do not in any way improve or increase the functioning powers of the digestive organs and they do not remove any of the causes of digestive impairment. On the contrary, the continued use of any one of them or all of them, without exception, further impairs the digestive powers.

The use of "digestive aids" and of means to "relieve" distress keeps the attention of the users directed away from the true solution of their problems and prevents them from learning the truth about their health and disease and how they may truly recover the former. That mankind has so long relied upon such measures, which have always failed, is a constant source of amazement to me. One expects even fools to learn from repeated experiences.

It is obvious to every intelligent reader of this book that a radically different approach to this subject is required if we are to successfully remedy indigestion. We gain nothing but added disease by enriching the manufacturers and distributors of drugs. These make millions out of substances that only add to the suffering of the poor deluded victims of the drug fetish. *Natural Hygiene* offers the people a real escape from their suffering and their bondage to ancient fallacies.

Good digestion is normal and when indigestion is present, it means that the powers of life have been reduced, usually by the conduct of the individual so suffering. After making due allowance for the effects of an unfavorable environment, we must ascribe most of the sufferings of men and women to the evil, though ignorant it may be, and systematic departure from organic laws in the general mode of life. The state of health is only to be maintained by a due observance of all the laws of life in their combination. How much more efficient is the process of digestion when food is taken in a serene and unexcited state of mind, compared with the working of the same process when food is taken in a state of mental agitation, from whatever source derived! And how greatly is the process of digestion affected by the conduct of the same person after meals, in relation to repose or work! Rest after eating is indispensable to good digestion. No man can digest his food well who does not half masticate it and who bolts from his dining table to his business like a greyhound slipped from the leash.

When life is lived at such a pace, as it often is in the larger cities, that everything, including eating, is done at breathless speed, when the jaws cannot masticate fast enough, and the food is gulped down half chewed, when the "eater" rushes immediately back to work without any rest whatever of body or mind, and this from day to day and from year to year, so long as the powers of life hold out, the Nemesis of outraged nature takes its toll. No man's capacity for continuing a galley-slave life is limitless, but capacity varies depending upon variations in the constitutional powers of different individuals. The stronger will hold out longer than his weaker brother, but sooner or later the most robust must succumb to the exhausting effects of such a life.

Whether through want or redundancy, through dissipation or over-exertion of any kind, when the human constitution becomes impaired and vitality fails, one of the first symptoms of the vital depression is an enfeeblement of the powers of digestion.

We have only to consider for a moment the many influences that certainly lessen the bodily vigor of man to realize that everybody in civilized society is more or less enervated. We may divide these influences roughly into *sins of commission* and *sins of omission*. Sins of omission may be said to be the offspring of ignorance of the laws of life or of willful neglect, or both. Sins of commission are those where the laws of life are not only wittingly neglected, but where they are positively and of purpose violated in the pursuit of either business or of pleasure. The same enervating influences may, perhaps, also be divided into those which are forced upon mankind by the necessities and struggles of life (by a socio-economic environment over which he, as an individual, has no control), and those which are adventitious, or in a manner, self-sought. The evils of the misery and poverty of the poorer classes are matched by those of the dissipations and enervating luxuries of the wealthy classes. Speculation, gambling and excitements of every kind make the largest drains on the nervous system. However, and from whence arising, whether from unavoidable over-toil of the mental and physical worker, or from the suicidal indulgence of the man of fashion, or from a combination of both these broad factors, the result is the same.

With the habitual violation of the laws of life, or more narrowly, with the habitual indulgence in enervating activities, the slow sapping of the energies of the constitution results in a progressive enervating of the body—a state of lowered nerve-energy not always recognized at first and the warnings not readily listened to—but as sure in its downward progress as the loosened avalanche. The result is the prostration of the bodily and mental powers and the degradation of the whole man.

Whenever, through a continual violation of the laws of life, the constitutional powers become enfeebled, not only is the excretory function greatly weakened, giving rise to toxemia (a state of poisoning by the retention of normal body waste), but also the digestive and assimilative powers become impoverished so that the nutrition of the body is lowered commensurate with the degree of constitutional enfeeblement. Indigestion follows with its consequent slow starving of the sufferer.

In such an enfeebled individual no change of diet can bring about a restoration of health until after all the causes of general enervation have been removed and sufficient rest has been secured to enable the body to restore its functioning activities. It should be obvious that if the power to digest and assimilate food is not increased, all attempts to "build-up" the patient by any kind of feeding program will prove abortive and useless. It is even more futile to attempt to restore digestive power by the use of drugs—tonics, astringents, barks, mineral acids, prepartions of iron, etc.—as these only further impair an already greatly impaired constitution and add to the digestive enfeeblement.

To substitute one source of enervation for another is not a rational procedure. To undertake to rest, while, at the same time, undergoing a whole series of palliating treatments—baths, massages, electrical treatments, adjustments, colonic irrigations, enemas, etc., —is to fail to achieve full health. Bear in mind that when you learn to live in conformity with the laws of life you will be forever delivered from the torture of the futile effort to destroy the necessary consequences of your misconduct. Only when we have learned to live within the confines of physiological and biological law can we transmute into a song of gladness that moan of pain and wail of despair that goes up from the earth today.

The intelligent person, viewing the great number of so-called diseases that arise out of this prostration of the functions of life, and realizing that they have one and all grown out of the habitual violations of the laws of life, will recognize at once that the first step in the restoration of health must needs be to make amends at once by an unconditional return to implicit and perfect obedience to the laws that have been so perseveringly violated. The patient, it should be evident, must be brought back to that completely healthful manner of life from which, alone, in its totality, we know that there is prospect of effecting a genuine restoration of health.

Is it possible to imagine a patient being rationally treated after a different manner? Can we conceive of a patient, while adhering steadfastly in his manner of life, to the identical habits which gave rise to his suffering, to be *cured* by drugs, or serums, or vaccines, or by surgery? Plainly it is impossible, unless, of course, we cast our physiology and, along with it, our common sense, to the four winds.

In the first place, the patient's nervous system, having been prostrated from overwork, over indulgence, stimulation (irritation), and excesses of many and varied kinds, it is plain that he must, above all things, have rest. Accordingly, we would order a peremptory release from all mental and bodily activities and duties that constitute a drain upon his energy resources. This is the *sine que none* of recovery. It is plain that, above all things, the enervated individual must have rest and this must include mental repose as well as bodily rest.

The physiological importance of repose of the mind to the performance of the function of digestion, on the healthy performance of which, as previously stated, vital results depend, explains the overriding importance which we have attached to the principle of nervous repose. Mental rest is best secured by a change of scenes from the haunts of business or pleasure, in the gas-laden atmosphere of the towns and cities, with their incessant noise and hubbub, to the delights of a quite country retreat in some picturesque district abounding in pleasant and varied scenery, with fresh breezes of health to play about the patient and over-head from morning to night, where he may enjoy the quiet repose of nature and bask in her healthful sunshine.

These patients discover that, in the long run, drugs do not answer the needs of their problem. On the contrary, they find themselves growing daily worse while resorting to drugs and resort to larger and larger doses, or to frequent changes of drugs. This progressive deterioration of function is due not alone to the impairing effects of the drugs, but also to the neglect of the original impairing causes, which the resort to drugs guarantees. It is hopeless to think of *curing* a disease while the manner of life that is the radical cause of all the trouble is persevered in.

The "two paths" of life are open to all alike. One leads to health, strength, happiness and longer life. It crowns us with honor and gives us a richer, fuller, more abundant life. The other leads as surely to disease, weakness, unhappiness and premature death as the cast stone falls back to earth. It crowns us with dishonor and gives us pains and an empty life. Which path will you follow? The choice is yours; nor can anyone else make the choice for you. Law and order are not respecters of persons and everyone will be rewarded or penalized according to the life he lives.

Are you dissipating or spending time and money on an abnormal appetite? What are your habits? Are they lawful (physiological) and such as you can expect good to flow from? Are you indulging in games of chance or in perverted practices? Are you certain that your mode of living—your mental and physical practices—conform with the laws of life? Keep in mind always that it is the right use of the body and mind that provides for man the best development and highest happiness.

Nor, can we approach the problem before us with any single factor solution. We are dealing with a state of affairs that has grown out of a varied assortment of antecedent factors and it can remedied only by duly considering each of these elemental causative factors. It is not enough to enjoin one enervating habit. All must be stopped at once and refrained from thereafter, if true success is to crown our efforts.

Just as the first step in the restoration of functioning power to the enfeebled organism is the discontinuance of all enfeebling practices, so the second step in the restoration of power to the enervated constitution is rational use of the combined materials and influences that constitute the *Hygienic System*. After all causes of enfeeblement have been removed, rest, sleep, food of the proper kind, exercise, fresh air, pure water, sunshine and healthful mental and moral influences are essential to the restoration of integrity of structure and efficiency of function.

When once, by *Hygienic* means, the body has been freed of its load of toxins, its nerve energy has been restored to normal, elimination has been re-established and the digestive and assimilative powers have been restored, there follows a gradual return to health. Until this has been done, the best of diets will not and cannot give the desired results. How many patients have sunk into their graves, in chronic as well as in acute disease, amid the strictest regulations of their diets, thus attesting the inefficacy of diet to preserve the sick and restore them to health, when disconnected from the series of appropriate hygienic materials and influences!

Hygienic factors are not of great importance in local treatment, but have their greatest, or sole value in their benefits to the whole organism. Thus, while food is of no value when applied locally, its value, when used by the whole body, is undisputed. Hence, as an indispensable basis of the work of the *Hygienist,* we must endeavor to secure to the patient the full benefit of all the *Hygienic* means, in their entire plentitude, for only thus can the patient be given a fair chance of recovery. Thus understood the phrase *Natural Hygiene* acquires a real significance, at once novel, startling, intense and delicious.

It is necessary to emphasize that food alone, important as it is in both health and disease, is not enough to assure either the preservation or the restoration of health. It is only in its physiological connection with water, exercise, rest, sleep and other elements of the *Hygienic System*, that its true value becomes manifest. Of these combined means, contributing severally to the remedial processes of the body, and each essential to these processes, it is enough to point out that it would be impossible to assign superior value to any over the rest, the simple fact being that each is indispensable, and that health is restored under the *Hygienic System* not by one *hygienic* factor alone, but through the combined remedial use of all of them.

It cannot be too strongly insisted upon, as a scientific fact, that it is the whole of the aforementioned hygienic factors, in their plenary combination and harmonious co-adaptation to the physiological wants of the living organism, which constitute the material and subtle means employed by the organism in the restoration of health. The natural or *Hygienic* care of the sick, made up, as it is, of so many concurrent and interdependent factors, cannot be held responsible for the failures that attend the unscientific and wholly one-sided application of some one or two hygienic elements by the ignorant and inexperienced.

Physiological rest—fasting—is of value in all forms of impaired health, but in indigestion it is a sure means of providing rest for an over-worked digestive system. In fasting practically all of the organs of the body reduce their activities, hence they rest. The exceptions are the organs of elimination (excretion) and these step up their activities; hence, during the fast the body is enabled to free itself of its accumulated load of toxic waste. The combination of mental, physical and physiological rest constitutes an ideal means of promoting elimination.

The fast should not be undertaken at home, where there are distractions, annoyances, and responsibilities and where friends and relatives interpose objections to it. It is best taken in a *Hygienic* institution under the supervision of an experienced *Hygienist*. In the *Hygienic* institution the patient is in a position, both physically and mentally, that makes it comparatively easy, not only to fast, but also to break bad habits. Here, too, is the place for him to cultivate and fix new and good habits. Indeed, it will always be best for the patient to remain in the institution until the new habits have become so much a part of him that he will experience little difficulty in continuing them once he has returned home. This is vitally important to continued progress in health and in preserving health, once this has been regained.

Let us not close our eyes to the obvious fact that health, when lost, can only be re-acquired by a laborious process in which the patient himself must play, by far, the principal role, and must faithfully and manfully carry out that fundamental truth in a systematic routine of healthful practices, till the end is achieved.

CHAPTER X

The Hygienic Institution

Originally it was the practice to call *Hygienic* institutions Hygeian Homes. At present the tendency is to call them Health Schools. They are called Health Schools for two reasons: First, the emphasis is placed on health in these establishments, rather than upon disease. Second, they are actually schools, where the patients are taught the simple natural ways of life that build and maintain health. They are taught to think and act in the language of health. It is the conviction of every true *Hygienist* that he has not done his full duty to his patients when he has piloted them back to health; his full duty has been done only when he has taught the patients how to remain healthy. The *Hygienist* is, therefore, a doctor in the true meaning of the term.

As it should be the prime aim of every enlightened man, in caring for the sick, to endeavor to provide for the patient the full benefit of all hygienic means, in their entire plenitude, as the indispensable basis of operations, the site of the *Hygienic* institution must be chosen because of its general salubrity, above all because of the purity and freshness of the air, the excellence of the water, the abundance of sunshine, and the fertility of the soil (for, upon the soil depends the quality of the foods fed to the patients).

Climate, too, is an important consideration. For the invalid, whether chronic or convalescing from an acute disease, there is always the South where the long-locked springs of life respond in free gushes to the melting, passionate aromas and gentle breezes of a warm clime, while they only trickle in the frost-bound climes of the North. In the land of the honeysuckle and the orange blossom, where gentle breezes from the Gulf give mild summers and cool summer nights, where warm winters make sunbathing possible throughout the winter season, the invalid may find renewal of life and increase of vigor.

But location is not all. A *Hygienic* institution is dedicated, wholly and solely, to purposes of health, and its internal arrangement and management is nicely and minutely adapted to this end. This requires system in the conduct of its program and it necessitates that the patient shall observe the few simple, healthful rules and practices of the institution.

A great advantage of being in the *Hygienic* institution is that the *Hygienist* has his patients almost always under his eyes—he is thus enabled to see that all the measures of hygienic care are attended to by the patients and attendants, in the most thoroughgoing manner. Moreover, being on the spot, he is in a position to discriminate with the utmost nicety the effects upon the patient of every item of care and of making whatever modifications in the plan of care that are required by the individual patient. This proves to be of the utmost benefit to the patient, and of great value to the *Hygienist* who is thus enabled to study at first hand, in a thoroughly scientific manner, his patients and their care. As his experience grows his services to his patients become more and more valuable.

The institution possesses other distinct advantages to the patient. First, every temptation is removed from out of his path. His friends and relatives are not around him urging him to continue on in his old mode of living. On the contrary, every one about him in the *Hygienic* institution encourages him in the work of breaking away from his disease inducing mode of living and in cultivating new and healthful habits. He is surrounded by good influences and is under the constant watchful eye of the doctor so that, under the combined influence of these factors, he is enabled to relinquish, in a short time, and with comparative ease to himself, a habit against which he would probably have struggled long and, perhaps, in vain while living in his own home with no support except the intermittent suggestions of his own unstable will.

The coffee and tea drinker, the tobacco user, the alcohol addict, the worrier, etc., is placed in a position, both physically and socially, that makes it comparatively easy to break off bad habits; habits that are very difficult to relinquish under ordinary circumstances and by the mere force of will. Indeed, the very hygienic regime, itself, often to the great surprise of the patient, makes the abandonment of bad habits comparatively easy. With physical and moral influences simultaneously at work, with the strong force of example all around him to assist his flagging will, being continually surrounded by other health-seekers, all of them struggling for the same prize, and more or less earnest in a course of well-doing, he is encouraged and buoyed up in his efforts. Success is certain. No one who has even a small understanding of human nature will undervalue such an influence for good.

To break old habits it is often necessary to dissociate oneself from the associations that have helped in their development and that continue to foster such habits. As a means of breaking up the associations under which faulty mental and physical habits have arisen and which are, to a great degree, responsible for the habits, a change of scenery and associations is often best. To the man of strength and determination, most of the unfavorable elements in his environment become just so many obstacles for him to hurdle. Unfortunately, men of strength and determination are not common.

And there is, in a general way, the great advantage to be derived from the discipline acquired by going through such a program—that of continually sacrificing luxuries and idle tastes and habits of every kind, of overcoming the antipathy, all too common even in health, to do that which, however advantageous to us, costs a determined and sustained effort. In this way it may be said that a period of *Hygienic* care is a moral no less than a physical gymnastic and it is quite certain that it is next to impossible to carry it out in its entirety except in an establishment dedicated exclusively to the purpose and organized in all respects in accordance with its requisites.

It may be well to speak, in this connection of the agreeableness, in a social sense, of the kind of life prevailing in a *Hygienic* institution, as a feature of undoubted import. Every one knows, from his own experience, the hygienic value of cheerful and easy society uncramped by the rules of false etiquette. To the invalid this is of special value. It lightens and brightens his way, and makes his work of recovery (and work it is) sit lightly on him. It keeps him in good spirits and prevents him from brooding over his own ailments.

The example of other patients, many of them worse than he is, recovering or recovered is truly of incalculable value to him, as it supplies him with a genuine basis of hope and encouragement. This is a benefit supplied by a *Hygienic* institution that is almost peculiar to the *Hygienic system*. If the institution is located in the country, as it should be, the quietness of the surroundings, the inspiring contact with nature, walks in the country, among the flowers and trees, the cheering songs of birds, and the many other agreeable things of country surroundings afford an advantage that is wholly lacking in the city or town.

A hospital is very far from good, even as regards the material treatment administered to the patients. It is much worse in a psychological sense, where everything concurs to aggravate the patient's troubles. Can anything be more desolate for a sick person than to be shut up in a ward of the hospital, with the dying and dead, breathing the foul air, hearing nothing but groans and complaints, attended by imperious mercenaries and treated like a slave? The hospital is for the sick what the alms-house is for the well-born poor; a succor which sinks him into the grave while he still lives.

I have indicated the many and various advantages to the patient of being in a *Hygienic* institution and I hope I have made these clearly intelligible. I need but add a few words about the efficacy and general applicability of *Hygienic* measures and processes in the care of the sick. *Hygienic* care is not based upon any notion of specifics but rests upon a totally different conception of the nature of disease and the requirements of recovery. Its rationale is based on the broad and distinctly characteristic principle that the living organism possesses within itself, in its original constitution, its own powers and means of restoration; that it is constantly endeavoring to work out its own recovery; that it frequently succeeds in its efforts without outside aid and that when its powers of self-healing are not sufficient to effect a restoration to health, the aid of the *Hygienist* must be founded on the primary laws of life as unfolded by biology and physiology. This means that our measures of care of the sick must be the identical means, variously modified, to meet the varying conditions of the sick, that are required for maintaining health. Our reliance, in other words, is on the natural agencies of health. Our cardinal remedial means are air, water, natural foods properly combined, rest (physical, mental, sensory and physiological), warmth, sunshine and healthful mental and moral influences. Together with these natural agencies of health, we must endeavor to find and remove all causes of disease from the life of the patient. These, then, are the tools with which the *Hygienist* works, and I for one can answer for their efficacy.

Principles of Natural Hygiene

By Herbert M. Shelton, N. D., as printed in
Dr. Shelton's Hygienic Review, 1949.

The Hygienic System not only introduced a *materia hygienica* and a new practice, but also a new theory and philosophy in biological science that is at variance with and in opposition to all the fundamental doctrines and dogmas on which all medical systems, past and present, have been founded. It claims to have ignored the false principles of the old schools (and of the new; and to have based its philosophy and its practice upon the unerring and demonstrable laws of nature. The principles and practices of the hygienic school are comparatively new, original and independent. They have never been written in medical books, nor taught in medical schools, nor recognized by the medical profession. While they are each and all in direct opposition to each and all of the fundamental principles on which the popular medical systems are based, they are demonstrably in harmony with the laws of nature.

The *Hygienic System* not only rejects wholly and totally, as both unnecessary and injurious, each and all of the poisons known to the *materia medicoas* of the medical schools as drug-remedies, but it also rejects the philosophy or theories on which their employment is predicated. *Hygiene* controverts all their fundamental dogmas, denies all their pretended science, challenges all of their philosophy, and condemns nearly all of their practices.

Let me begin by defining my subject. *Hygiene* is that branch of biology which investigates and applies the conditions upon which life and health depend, and the means by which health is sustained in all its virtue and purity, and restored when it has been lost. *Hygiene* is not a system of therapeutics. It professes to build health in all forms of diseased states by the employment of hygienic agents alone and without the employment of poisons or resort to enervating palliatives of any nature. Constructive surgery forms the only non-hygienic measure ever endorsed by the natural hygienist.

A true hygiene is not empirical, but rests upon the immutable and unchanging laws of nature. All real science comes from recognition of the laws of nature. These are the principles which embody all truth, and whose proper arrangement into a system constitutes all science, and art is but the application of these truths to uses, to the production of the desired results.

The laws of nature, the truths of the universe, the principles of science, are just as certain, as fixed and immutable in their relations to human organization, in relation to life, in relation to health, in relation to happiness, in relation to disease, as they are in relation to all things else.

Because man has not studied himself aright he knows not the laws of his own being. Instead of looking to the laws of nature for enlightenment he has gone in pursuit of strange gods, and become the worshipper of idols, and the victim of his own folly. He has sought to understand the ways of evil instead of good, he has studied the "laws of disease" rather than the philosophy of health, he has seated disorder on the throne of the universe, and in trying to adapt himself to this king, he has been led into a thousand foolish fashions, perpetrated innumerable violations of the laws of order, and brought upon himself inconceivable miseries so that we may say of mankind personified:

"Sickness sits caverned in his hollow eye."

Health is nothing more than life in a normal state because of normal conditions; while disease is life in an abnormal state because of abnormal conditions. Here is a very simple, but entirely correct definition of disease; it is abnormal vital action.

What is necessary to the production of a living thing is also necessary to its preservation. The human body is developed under certain natural conditions and influences, and by the use of certain natural agents and materials, and these same conditions and influences and materials are essential and all that are essential to its maintenance in a state of health. What causes a human being to grow into manhood or womanhood in health and vigor is necessary to preserve that health and vigor, and all that is necessary.

A rational hygienist will study and understand exactly and precisely the nature and influences of air, water, food, light, exercise, rest, sleep, temperature, clothing, housing, noise, the emotions, etc., and apply the knowledge daily, hourly, constantly, acting ever and always in proper relation to the laws of life, to the preservation and restoration of health. What is needed is a complete system of hygiene, not an exaggerated attention given to but one hygienic factor. Not exercise alone, not diet alone, not sunshine alone, not emotional poise alone, not any one factor alone: but a well-rounded, correlated and integrated system, which includes all the conditions and materials of healthy life. Health must be built and maintained as a unit and must rest upon the total mode of living.

In its widest sense, hygiene is the application of the principles of nature to the preservation and restoration of health. Applied to the sick, it consists in finding the cause of the patient's suffering and removing this, and in restoring to the patient the conditions of a healthy life. This is accomplished by teaching him how to prepare and eat a proper diet, secure abundance of fresh air, to use sunshine properly, how to exercise, rest, clothe himself properly, etc. It may be said to be a system of purification, vivification and rejuvenation. By the use of agents and conditions that are normal to the body, the system is cleansed, invigorated and restored to healthy action.

Health and disease are not accidents, but developments of law. Just as the same law of gravity carries a balloon upward under one set of conditions and brings it back to earth under another, or floats a ship under one set of conditions and sinks it under another, just as it is the same chemical affinity that preserves a stick of dynamite under one set of conditions and explodes it under another, so the same law of life produces health under one set of conditions and disease under another. A knowledge of the laws of life makes health and disease matters of our own choice. We can have the one or the other as we supply the conditions for the one or the other.

The *Hygienic System* was the first and, so far, the only school that makes the laws of nature and the conditions of health its chief reliance in the preservation and restoration of health. These are taught in no other school on earth save the *Hygienic*. Nor are they proclaimed to be taught in any other. On these points, we speak advisedly. For three thousand years medical men, philosophers and scientists of the highest abilities have sought an understanding of the -essential nature of disease, the mode of action of drugs, the precise relation of drugs to disease and the healing power of nature. Today disease is listed as one of the "seven modern mysteries." Most of the standard works on pharmacology contain brief efforts at explaining the *modus operandi* of drug action, but none of these are satisfactory. How drugs act is still as much a mystery as the nature of disease itself. No one pretends to understand the relation of drugs to disease: there seems to be little understanding of the healing power of nature and disease and the healing-powers are still, as they were in the days of Hippocrates, thought of as antagonistic forces or processes.

Confessing that they do not know the essential nature of any disease, medical men are incessantly drugging all disease, as though they know all about it. Confessing their lack of knowledge of the *modus operandi* of any drug they are incessantly using thousands of them as though the actions of all of them are known.

How can a successful means of dealing with anything be devised when the thing is not understood? If they do not know the essence of

disease and do not understand its nature, how can they build a successful method of treating the sick? A knowledge of the essential nature of
disease must be at the very foundation of any truly scientific care of
the sick. To attempt to operate a locomotive, while one is unacquainted
with the power of steam, would be rash; but to treat sick people, while
ignorant of the nature and cause of disease, as medical men acknowledge
they are, is madness, even to insanity. He who cannot make one blade of
grass to grow may destroy millions.

Now *Hygienists* do profess to understand the nature of disease and
the apparent actions of drugs, and understanding these things they
reject all drugs.

Disease is as much a vital process as is health. Health is vital action
in the construction and conservation of bodily organs, and disease is
vital action in defense and reparation of the same organs. Health is the
normal play of all the vital functions, disease is remedial effort, or their
abnormal play. The difference between health and disease is simply this:
Health is the regular and normal performance of the functions of the
body; it is normal action — physiology; disease is irregular and abnormal action — pathology. Health expresses the aggregate of vital actions
and processes that nourish and develop the body and all its organs and
structures and provide for reproduction; in other words, health is the
action of the vital powers in building up and replenishing the organic
structures; or in still plainer words, the conversion of the elements
of food into the elements of the body's tissues, and the elimination of
waste. Disease is the aggregate of vital actions and processes by which
poisons are expelled and damages repaired; it is the action of the same
powers that are active in health, in defending the organism against
injurious or abnormal agencies and conditions.

To illustrate these two principles; the body does not act upon alcohol
as it does upon food. It digests, absorbs, circulates, assimilates and
uses food. It does not digest and assimilate alcohol. Alcohol is absorbed
and circulated, but it is not appropriated. It is not used. The body acts
against it, to resist it, to expel it, as it does all other poisons. The normal
work of digesting food is healthy action; the abnormal work of resisting
and expelling alcohol is diseased action.

And thus the healing power of nature, the nature of which has been
sought since the days of Hippocrates, and disease turn out to be one
and the same thing. A partial recognition of this fact is implied in
the belated admission by pathologists, of the constructive character
of inflammation and the beneficial character of fever. The healing
principle is always in the living system itself. All living organisms are
self-constructing, self-defending and self-repairing. The only power

that can heal is the power that repairs; the only power that can repair is the power that produces; the power that now produces, repairs, heals, etc., is the power that is originally produced. The power that evolved a full-grown man from a fertilized ovum is the only healing power. It is an intrinsic, not an extrinsic power. The power that produced the organism is in it to maintain it.

The power which brought us into being, which causes us to grow through the various stages of development to manhood or womanhood, also repairs the organism, sustains its growth, performs its functions, heals its lesions — in a word, this power constitutes the only healing, repairing, preserving force. Huxley's "Hidden Artist," that made and fashioned the organs and the organism, is always on hand to continue its work in growth and repair and in function. In every living organism the process of repair is the process of reproduction, the same power which brought it into existence; is the same power that performs all the functions of life. It is folly to think some outside power can perform the functions of life.

It is by cell reproduction that repair takes place and this is not the work of any extrinsic agent or force, but of the inherent, intrinsic power of life. Nobody doubts that it is the same power that brought us into being that heals in the case of a wound. A surgeon would not think of opening the abdomen of a patient, if he was not certain that the processes of life would heal the wound thus inflicted. For he knows that he possesses no curative agencies that can heal a wound. Just why we insist upon thinking that some other agency than that of the powers of life are requisite in the healing of disease, in those cases where the causes of the trouble are not obvious, is hard to explain.

Healing is a process of evolution just as birth, growth and development are. Neither medicines, water, food, exercise, nor anything else external to the organism have any healing power. The same power that brought a man into health keeps him in health, and it alone can restore him to health. That power resides in the man, and nowhere else in nature. The same powers and processes of life are in operation in disease as in health. In disease, no new or extra-vital power is superadded to the processes of life.

Let me now explain the apparent actions of drugs. Observations of the phenomena that follow the use of a drug demonstrate that certain effects follow. But why they follow, how they follow, and what is their real cause, as distinct from their occasion, have not been determined. Until we know what cause produces a given effect we cannot explain the effect. As nobody has ever explained how drugs act on the body we offer this opposite explanation—that the living system acts on the drug. On the basis of this theory we find the explanation of most of the so-called effects of drugs and, we believe, that in time, all the other so-called actions will be explained on this basis. Whatever principle will explain the *modus operandi* of one poison will explain the *modus operandi* of them all.

We find the explanation of what are mistakenly called the actions of drugs in the laws of organization — in physiology rather than in chemistry or physics. Life and its variable phenomena furnish the proper field of inquiry. On the basis of such investigations we deny that drugs act at all, but insist that as lifeless, inorganic substances, they are as passive, inert, quiescent, and inactive when taken into the body as when resting in their various bottles on the druggist's shelves. They are acted upon, but do not act.

The *Hygienic* philosophy reduces this mysterious problem to a single truism, by reference to the primary premise — the law of relation between organic and inorganic matter. The law that applies to this problem is that in the relations between living and lifeless matter, living matter is active, lifeless matter is passive always. Medicines do not act at all. Lifeless matter, we reiterate, does not act on the living. This is the universal law in the relations of the living organism to everything that surrounds it. The drug in the stomach, the poison in the blood, the 'medicine' in the drug store, the food on the table, the water in the pitcher — these are all passive in their relations to the living organism. The organism acts upon all these things, either to appropriate them or to reject them and expel them. Drugs are lifeless, inorganic, inert substances and have no relation to the living save that of inertia, the same as a dry stick or a- stone and since the incapacity to act is an inseparable characteristic of all lifeless matter, while, on the other hand, action is an inseparable characteristic of life, we know that whenever action takes place between living and lifeless matter, the former and not the latter, does the acting; they do nothing. They are done unto. They are acted upon. The living thing is active and the lifeless thing is passive. This is no denial of the mechanical actions of masses of matter, nor of the chemical actions of atoms of matter. We deny only that drugs have the actions — physiological, medicinal, etc. — attributed to them by pharmacologists and physicians.

Our main position, in general terms, may be thus stated: The symptoms or phenomena which result when a drug-remedy is taken into the system are the evidences of vital resistance to the drug (the action of the system against the drug contemplating its expulsion) and are not evidences of the remedial action of the drug on the body, as is commonly supposed. The law can be demonstrated and we think that it may be best expressed about as follows: *The resident forces in the various tissues, acting preservatively, give rise to all the phenomena that are mistaken for the actions of drugs.* It is *modus operandi* of the living organism. The *modus operandi* of drugs is a misnomer. On the basis of the various medical theories that have been offered to account for "drug action," it is impossible to give the rationale of the "action" of any drug. On the *Hygienic* theory it is possible to explain the rationale of all of them. The rationale of the effects of all "medicines" is inseparably connected with life. Whatever will explain the *modus operandi* of one "medicine" or one poison will explain the *modus operandi* of all of them. Two separate and distinct principles of action are not admissible.

This is either true or false. If true, the whole system of administering drugs to cure disease ought to be abandoned as unsound in science and injurious in results. All drug remedies are absolutely poisonous. This difference of principle involves the essential philosophy of drug medication in all its schools, modes, phases, and modifications. The point on which we differ comes to the veritable explanation, the rationale, of all remedial or medicinal agents.

Medical men in all ages have mistaken the actions of the living organism in self-defense for the actions of foreign substances upon it. They have mistaken the vital action in expelling foreign substances from the body for an attack of some outside entity upon the body. In thus mistaking the true nature of operations seen in disease, they have attempted to subdue, suppress and destroy the very actions and processes that alone can save the life of the patient. In their efforts to cure (exorcise or kill an imaginary enemy) they have been warring upon the human constitution. All the importance attached to the management of the sick with drugs comes from a non-recognition of these principles, from a mistake in regard to the essential nature of the actions that follow the taking of poisons.

The philosophy of *Hygienic* care of the sick is predicated on the primary premise that those things which are constitutionally adapted to the preservation of health are also the proper things to use in restoring health. The same agents and conditions that have been found necessary to the enjoyment of health are also best calculated to enable the body to overcome and remove unhealthy conditions within.

All healing power is inherent in the living organism and all true remedial agents (materials, influences, processes) must harmonize with the laws of life and must be susceptible of constructive use by the organism. No substance can be used remedially which bears no normal relation to the organism. All the "remedial agents" have normal or physiological relations to the living organism. They may be used constructively to preserve health, or remedially to restore health, but they are not cures. They may be abused and that abuse causes disease.

In the class of *Hygienic* agencies can be included only the actual necessities of life — food, air, water, sunlight, rest, sleep, relaxation, exercise, play, warmth, cleanliness, hope, faith, courage — and the means of securing these. For three thousand years these were classed as non-naturals. They were either rejected entirely or ignored in practice. Drugs were classed as naturals.

None of the real *Hygienic* materials and conditions can be dispensed with permanently. Such is the inherent nature of the truly *Hygienic* factors that their employment affords an actual compensation for the energy expended in their appropriation by the organism; a truly *Hygienic* agent and influence gives and does not merely take. Rightly used it gives more than it takes. Only when abused does it take more than it gives.

All too many people think of *Hygienic* agencies and conditions as limited in their work to the preservation of health. They think that, while *Hygiene* is good for the person in health, it is weak and unreliable in a state of sickness. When sick we need more potent, more powerful "remedies" — poisons — that in health we do not need. In fact, it is well-known that if a healthy person takes poison it will make him sick. We have, here, a strange perversion of truth and a strange anomaly of logic. Things that are good for the healthy are not good for the sick; things that are bad for the healthy are good for the sick.

Hygienists reject poisons. Indeed, the *Hygienists* are the only ones who have persistently and consistently rejected all poisons. Are poisons, then, *Hygienic* agencies? To believe in the necessity of any substance, or condition, we must have evidence that these are beneficial if used habitually in a state of health, that their use will effect some necessary result in a state of health. They must be indispensable to life. If drugs are *Hygienic* agencies they are actual necessities of life and their uses are not to be confined to times of illness alone. They are essential in health as well as in disease. To believe that they are *Hygienic* factors, we must believe that they are essential to effecting some necessary result in a state of health, and to regard them as *Hygienic* agents we must believe that the habitual use of them by a person in health would be beneficial.

Everything is poisonous which the system rebels against and rejects in a state of health. Everything is *Hygienic* which it seeks, uses and appropriates. Drugs are non-usable substances; they do not nourish the tissues, they cannot be transformed into blood and tissue, they cannot invigorate the body or any part of it, they cannot be used in any manner in the performance of any of the normal functions of life, nor in the performance of any of the abnormal actions of life, hence they must be expelled. They can only occasion vital resistance, hence their use results in a waste of vital power. They are definitely un-*hygienic* and opposed to all the vital interests of life.

Science gives us no grounds for including poisonous agents among *Hygienic* agents. No one supposes that poisons (drugs) are necessary in a state of health, that they are necessities of life, or that their use produces any necessary or beneficial result in a state of health. Drugs (and many other agents) employed in the treatment of the sick have nothing in their nature that can afford any compensation to the organism for the energy employed in resisting and expelling them. It is only in a state of impaired health that their use is supposed to be needed. But if poisons cannot be beneficial in a state of health, they cannot be helpful in a state of sickness. If all truly remedial agents have normal or physiological relations to the living organism, as *Hygienists* proclaim, then drugs of every kind cannot be classed as "remedial agents."

Should the sick be poisoned? That is a startling question. If our people had not been so badly miseducated this question could be answered by asking: should the well be poisoned? For there is no more reason why a sick man should be poisoned than a well man. No physician has ever been able to give a rational theory, or even a plausible hypothesis, or even the shadow of a shade of an argument, why any person, because he is sick, should take into his body a poison that would certainly induce disease in a well person.

Everybody seems to know that drug-medicines are poisons; that they are always injurious to persons in health. All persons are very careful to exclude them from their victuals and drink. They seem to be aware that if, by accident or design, they take them into the system while it is in health, sickness will be the consequence. What person would dare to take an ordinary dose of calomel, or antimony while in perfect health? Yet, let him get sick, and he swallows them, not only without fear, but as the essential conditions of safety. We suspect, indeed, we know, there is a terrible delusion abroad on this subject.

It is a strange practice that a remedy which always tends to kill is chosen to cure the sick. If poison be both our bane and our boon, we are indeed strangely made. In the days when physicians bled patients to cure them and butchers bled pigs to kill them, and gave arsenic to patients to cure them, while farmers fed arsenic to rats to kill them, a sick rat might refuse to eat arsenic because it kills well rats, but a sick man could not exercise so much intelligence.

It is not true that things which are poisonous in health become innocuous in disease. Nothing changes its relation to the human organism because this is sick or well. A food or a poison is so once and always— under all possible circumstances. Bread will never corrode the tissues and calomel will never nourish them, be the conditions of health or the circumstances of disease what they may.

The idea of poisoning a person because he is sick is founded on a false notion of the nature of disease. Disease is regarded, in all teachings of the medical books, as a something foreign to the organism, as an enemy; and poisons are given to war upon and destroy the enemy. But as the truth happens to be the exact contrary, all this poisoning business happens to be exactly wrong—nothing more nor less than a war on human constitutions.

There are better ways of caring for the sick than that of poisoning them. They need helpful, not hurtful things. It will amaze the uninitiated to watch the body and see what it can do for itself in the way of recovery if left uncrippled by drugs of any kind, in large or small doses.

History reveals to us that the theory that the earth revolves on its axis was controverted for twelve hundred years before it was finally accepted. It was so preposterous and absurd to the people who knew that the earth is flat and that the sun goes under and around the earth once in twenty-four hours, that they could not accept it. In like manner, it is difficult to get people to accept the simple truism that *Hygienic* agents, chat is, agents adapted to health, are better for the sick than pathogenic agents, that is, agents that induce sickness in the well.

Getting along in sickness without drugs of some kind has a strange sound to most of us when we first hear of it. The idea of caring for the sick with poisons has become deeply ingrained in us. Most of us are "born with it." It has grown with our growth and strengthened with our strength. It has been associated with all our thoughts, observations and experiences on the subject of caring for the sick. This is the reason that we must be in some measure, at least, un-educated and re-educated. Getting along without drugs may seem as preposterous as did the theory that the earth rotates on its axis and revolves around the sun, to the ancient astronomers. Yet some of the most remarkable recoveries on record have occurred without medical treatment of any kind. The great error of physicians has been that of attributing recovery to the operations of their poisons, while they have left out of account the healing powers of the body itself.

Hygienists are not engaged in curing disease. Indeed, we hold that ill efforts to cure disease are based upon false notions of the essential nature of disease.

Disease is a process of purification and reparation. It is not an enemy of the vital powers but a struggle of the vital powers themselves in self-defense. We of the *Hygienic* school do not regard the diseases which are said to kill so many every year as of themselves, dangerous; we hold that the great mortality seen in these diseases is due to suppressive and combative treatment. Disease is not a thing to be removed, expelled, subdued, broken up, destroyed, conquered, or cured or killed. It is not a thing, but an action; not an entity, but a process; not an enemy at war with the living organism, but a remedial effort; not a substance to be opposed, but an action to be cooperated with.

The *Hygienic System* is not a collection of therapies and cures. Nor are *Hygienists* engaged in a ceaseless search after new, more novel, ever more sensational, and miraculous cures. In the whole history of the *Hygienic* movement, not a single one of its practitioners has brought forth a single cure., No rapid succession of wonder-cures from *Hygienic* sources, each to enjoy its brief day in the sun, only to pass into that long night that is followed by no sunrise. *Hygienists* go all the way in the matter. We have no "curative agencies" and recognize none. Disease the result of violation of physiological law and a return to obedience the condition of recovery.

Why experiment with a host of "remedies?" Why not study cause and effect? Only by removing the causes that have impaired the functions of life can a normal function be restored. This requires, first of e a full and thorough correction of the habits and conditions of life.

The principles of the *Hygienic System* are true, hence, if they a understood they will be believed; and if they are intelligently believe they will be successfully practiced; for the whole of *Hygienic* art, both in health and sickness, is merely the application of scientific principle to the varying circumstances of life, (of health and disease) and, sickness, to the constantly changing conditions of the patient. *Hygienic* methods are not empirical, they are not experimental, they are not hazardous and they are not to be employed haphazardly. The *Hygienic System* is established upon a settled and scientific basis, having fixed principles to guide the employment of all of its measures. Every particular process must conform to the principles of the system and all results are the results of unvarying accuracy.

The present much ado about psychosomatic medicine and about treating the whole man, the patient, instead of the disease is not new to *Hygienists*. We approach the matter from an entirely different angle than that of the physician and pseudo-psychologist, but caring for the whole man has been *Hygienic* practice from its beginning. Over a hundred years ago Sylvester Graham wrote: "If we could correctly understand the science of physiology or pathology, we must take into view and thoroughly investigate, the whole nature and condition and relation of man—he who treats of the functions of the human organs, and the diseases of the human body, without fully and accurately considering the modifying influences of the mind, and of the various physical and moral circumstances acting on the healthy and on the morbid sensibilities and sympathies of the system, may indeed form a theory which will have its day of popular acceptance, but fortunate without a parallel will it be, if it does not, sooner or later, prove to possess sufficient error to sink it into utter disrepute, if not total oblivion."

The pioneer *Hygienists* held that the "physical, mental, moral and spiritual" parts of man are "parts of one stupendous whole, of one grand personality." They said very forcefully that the *Hygienist* must not look only to physical health, but that the "mental, moral and spiritual health of the individual, of the collective man," is his legitimate scope. Resorting to scriptural phraseology, which the earlier *Hygienists* frequently did they pointed out that the physical, mental, moral and spiritual phases of man are all "members of one another," and that "if one member suffers all the members suffer with it, or if one member be honored, all the members rejoice with it."

For full health a complete and well-rounded program of physiological and biological living is essential. Health can only be produced as a unit and the total health program must meet all of the needs of life.

We are beginning to inquire, not how shall we get well, but, how shall we keep well. This is a wholesome change in public attitude towards health which has resulted directly from the work of the *Hygienists*. As important as *Hygienic* principles may be in giving the world better methods of caring for the sick, this is not the greatest benefit they are destined to confer upon the race. Far more important is their influence in preventing disease. An appreciation of *Hygienic* principles results in the understanding that in order to preserve health, the causes of disease must be avoided. This implies living in conformity with organic law and in all things, "cease to do evil and learn to do good."

Economy alone should cause people to adopt the *Hygienic System*. Its universal adoption by the people of the United States would save in physicians' bills, nursing bills, hospital bills, etc., alone, several hundred millions of dollars a year. An equal sum would be saved by avoiding loss of time from work or business. The enormous tax burden that the people bear to maintain public health organizations would be lifted from their shoulders. This enormous saving of money is small compared to the saving from suffering its adoption would assure.

Health is pre-eminently the great want of the age. A precise, intimate and practical knowledge of its conditions, and of the circumstances which induce disease, as well as of the way to remove diseases without incurring other evils as great, or worse, is the great need of the people. We believe the physical salvation of the human race depends on it.

As we understand the ways of nature and man, and the ways of man toward himself, all those examples of abnormal activity called disease and all premature deaths not caused by violence, are due to habits and practices perfectly explainable and as perfectly avoidable. And so believing, we cannot feel nor think that the physician, practitioner or *Hygienist* has performed his whole duty in merely acting as a "medical" adviser or treater of disease at the bedside of the sick and dying. He should at all times, be a teacher engaged in teaching the people how to live to avoid disease. This means that he should seek to make his services dispensable.

A true science of disease prevention, or of health building can rest upon correct principles only and these were discovered by *Hygienists*. What do these discoveries imply in practice? What principle did they establish in the healing art? Simply obedience to the laws of life. We cannot depart from them without incurring sickness. We cannot live in disobedience thereunto without perpetuating disease. Is there anything so strange, so astonishing in the proposition that the sick, in order to regain health, should obey the laws of life, just as much as should the well to preserve it? And yet, almost the whole world behaves in accordance with the ridiculous and incomprehensible muddle of medical men, that wholesome things are only adapted to the state of health, while unwholesome things are necessary for the conditions of disease.

These principles teach us plainly that a life which secures the greatest amount of bodily and mental vigor, which insures the longest period of earthly existence, which promotes the highest earthly happiness, and gives the utmost ability to do good in the world is only to be realized in the proper use of all things of earth and the abuse of none. Thus the *Hygienic* school supplies the strongest incentive which can be offered men, women and children to be "temperate in all things."

It is much easier to be well than sick. All nature is pledged to the maintenance and recovery of health. Health comes of itself, but we are in great pains to get our diseases. The elements of an unbounded success are wrapped up in the doctrine of health by healthful living. The statement of Dr. H. Lahn that the best medicine in all climates is a natural mode of living, may be changed to read: the best prophylactic in all climates is a natural mode of living.

It is much easier to keep the body in health than it is to restore it to health once it has become impaired. It is much easier to keep from developing bad habits than it is to break these habits after they have become fixed. How much better, then, to study *Hygiene* and use it to preserve health, than to study the intricacies and mysteries of *materia medica* and endeavor to restore health after it has been lost.

Our lives are so out of line with nature and our habits of thinking are in such perfect conformability with our lives, that we rarely conceive of the health and happiness that may be ours by a simple return to a normal mode of living. The ways of nature are not those of convention. We have strayed far from the paths of nature; so far indeed, that the ways of nature seem foreign to us. As a consequence, a "pernicious malady" is spreading among people and individuals, sapping them of physical and mental fiber. Until this malady is checked or remedied there can be no assurance of permanent health. The remedy will not be found in the realm of scientific research nor laboratory experiment. It can be found only when the people give up their unnatural ways and adjust themselves to the ways of nature.

Marvelously simple are all the works of nature; all the operations of her laws. To our perverted instincts and miseducated senses all may be complexity and confusion. The man who is himself in false relations to everything else will pronounce the whole universe to be chaos. The person who is in harmony with all other objects will find order, beauty, happiness everywhere.

Wonderfully plain are all the teachings of the ever-open volume of nature's book. Every page tells us of the laws of life, the conditions of health, the essentials of a better individuality, of a higher personality. All that we call good, and everything we term evil, are equally our guides and teachers. They lead us in the way we should go, or punish us when we are in the way we should not go, and compel us, as it were, to fulfill the design of nature.

Our present health, our earthly happiness, our personal development, our usefulness to others, our influence on the generations yet unborn, depend on the knowledge of a few exceedingly simple conditions, and our observance of them.

These *Hygienists* have endeavored for over a hundred years to teach the people. We have taught that health is the normal condition of the Human race. We have explained the way in which it is to be attained and preserved. Thousands have adopted our principles, and, in their lives, demonstrated their truthfulness and utility. But many more thousands there are who have never heard of them, or who have not that thorough understanding of the subjects they involve, which enables them to make, under all the varied circumstances of life the proper application.

It is indeed no small task to eradicate from society the accumulated errors of three thousand years; to convince the people of the utter fallacy of the popular medical system; to explode all of its false philosophy; to clear the ground of the rubbish of ages, and build up a new, a different, an independent medical science and healing art. But it must be done. It will be done.

These principles have a direct bearing upon the morals of the individual and of society. All good men will be better men by living in obedience to physiological law and thus enjoying good health; conversely, a bad man will be a worse man precisely in the ratio that he departs from the laws of his being in his voluntary habits. There is, in our judgment, a natural and determinate relation between internal conditions and outward conduct.

In medicine and religion poisons and penances take the place of truth and righteousness. Physicians profess to have provided man with means of escaping the natural and inevitable consequences of his conduct. Why, therefore, seek to know the right and do it? Why be good when you can buy absolution? Why avoid the causes of disease when you may be immunized against them? Why search for causes when a pill will set everything right? Why avoid injurious practices, when penicillin will erase their consequences? Why live cleanly when vaccines can make unclean living safe? Why behave lawfully when a sermon or a pill can annul the laws of life? Why think of consequences when we can beg, buy, borrow or steal a cure?

The physician, perhaps innocently because by his professional deeds, ignorantly acts as an abetter of vice, and perhaps crime, by professing to show how to escape by medical penance from the consequences of violations of the laws of life. By the mystical contents of his materia medica, by professional legerdemain, he professes to be able to counteract the operations of the laws of nature. He virtually proposes to the weak-minded inducements for violation of the laws of their being. Thus he leads the human race on to its deterioration. The absurdity, even the wickedness, of such a practice is apparent to all who will bestow a little thought upon it. If such things were really possible they would demoralize the race; for they would automatically license us to do wrong.

Teach men that nature's laws can be broken at pleasure, and mended when convenient; that they can violate all the laws of their being, and find immediate advantage or enjoyment in so doing, and then, when the consequences have become very grievous, they can resort to remedies to restore them to their former state of health, and they will do just what the majority of people the world over are led to do by their medical advisers — they will go on living in utter recklessness of nature's laws, incurring all manners of diseases, and employing physicians and "healers" of various kinds to dose away and treat away the inevitable consequences of their reckless follies. These doctrines of the shaman are the most demoralizing doctrines that have ever been entertained by the human mind.

Hygienists assert that, the world's redemption from disease, doctors, and drugs, depends on a practical recognition of the doctrine that nature's laws cannot be violated with impunity; that penalties will not be remitted; that nature has not provided remedies; that if wrong is done, evil consequences will follow; that every poisonous drug, and every unphysiological habit, and every unhealthful act, will make its injurious mark irreparably and forever; that our life, our strength, our health, will be measured exactly by our observance of organic law. This is a statement of a vital truth, the full realization of which, by the people as a whole, will lead inevitably to a revolution in their various modes of living. For the beginning of *Hygienic* wisdom is to "cease to do evil." It will be easy thereafter to "learn to do good."

Health and disease are according to obedience and disobedience. If wrong is done, evil consequences must follow. There are great errors in our habits of life, as evidenced by the great amount of faulty development, sickness and premature dying among us. But we cannot wipe these errors out with drugs, vaccines, serums, gland extracts, and the surgeon's knife. Nor can we ignore the errors of life. To teach that drugs are better than obedience and that the pathological products of animal sacrifices are better than conformity with the laws of life, is to completely demoralize all who accept and believe such doctrines. It is folly to think that consequences can be dosed or vaccinated away. Nature has made no provision to nullify nor destroy her own laws. The only real cure is a return to obedience. Nature does not bribe us to sin by promising us absolution. She does not hold out to us any hope that we may escape the consequences or effects of our unphysiological conduct by resort to any immunizing agent. There is no basis in all nature for the doctrine of immunization. Immunity, were it real, would mean the suspension of the law of cause and effect.

The best, indeed the only, method of promoting individual and public health is to teach people the laws of nature and thus teach them how to preserve their health. Immunization programs are futile and based on the delusion that the law of cause and effect can be annulled. Vaccines and serums are employed as substitutes for right living; they are intended to supplant obedience to the laws of life. Such programs are slaps in the face of law and order. Belief in immunization is a form of delusional insanity.

Obliterate these false doctrines of cure and immunization from medical schools, and books, teach the people the simple truth in relation to the nature of disease, the *modus operandi* of so-called remedies, and the theory of stimulation, and we shall have gone a long way towards the physical regeneration of the people.

Teach this generation the true relations between living and lifeless matter and the next generation will sing the song of a new redemption. Teach men and women to prevent disease by avoiding its causes rather than to attempt to cure it by administering the causes of other diseases and health and happiness will abound everywhere. If the people can be thoroughly indoctrinated with the principles of physiology and *Hygiene,* they will have very little need of physicians; and when they understand the nature of disease and the *modus operandi of* medicines, they will never consent to be poisoned because they are sick.

We are convinced that mankind can be educated in correct principles and trained in right practices so that sickness will cease to trouble us. It is our business to teach people how to prevent disease and not merely how to care for themselves when ill. We are not content to be mere tinkers and patchworkers. We are fully convinced also that the old medical systems and the present trends in medicine have mankind headed in the wrong direction.

I am well aware of the revolutionary character of the principles I have presented. I know that their acceptance by the public will work great changes, not only in the care of the sick and in the prevention of disease, but in many other fields of modern activity, but I am convinced that the physical salvation of our race depends upon their acceptance.

CPSIA information can be obtained
at www.ICGtesting.com
Printed in the USA
BVHW070713060822
643966BV00008B/1267